Register Now for Online Access to Your Book!

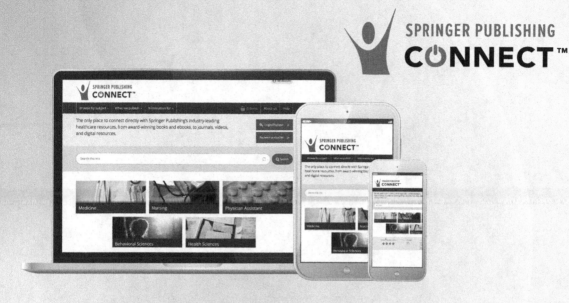

SPRINGER PUBLISHING
CONNECT™

Your print purchase of *Assisted Living Administration and Management Review* **includes online access to the contents of your book**—increasing accessibility, portability, and searchability!

Access today at:
http://connect.springerpub.com/content/book/978-0-8261-6735-4
or scan the QR code at the right with your smartphone. Log in or register, then click "Redeem a voucher" and use the code below.

> **VAA9KAYT**

Scan here for quick access.

Having trouble redeeming a voucher code?
Go to https://connect.springerpub.com/redeeming-voucher-code

If you are experiencing problems accessing the digital component of this product, please contact our customer service department at cs@springerpub.com

The online access with your print purchase is available at the publisher's discretion and may be removed at any time without notice.

Publisher's Note: New and used products purchased from third-party sellers are not guaranteed for quality, authenticity, or access to any included digital components.

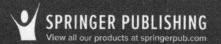

SPRINGER PUBLISHING
View all our products at springerpub.com

ASSISTED LIVING ADMINISTRATION AND MANAGEMENT REVIEW

Darlene Yee-Melichar, EdD, FGSA, FAGHE, is a professor and coordinator of gerontology at San Francisco State University (SF State) where she also serves as director of long-term care administration. She is the recipient of numerous awards and honors for her teaching excellence and service contributions to the campus, community, and profession.

Dr. Yee-Melichar's research interests in healthy aging, long-term care administration, minority women's health, and safety research and education are reflected in the six books, 109 journal articles, book chapters, book reviews, and technical reports she has written and the numerous professional and scholarly presentations she has made. She was active on the National Institutes of Health (NIH) Advisory Committee for Research on Women's Health, NIH Review Committee for Research Enhancement Awards Program, and Agency for Healthcare Research and Quality (AHRQ) special emphasis panels on Translating Research into Practice and Health Research Dissemination.

She chaired the U.S. Department of Health and Human Services (DHHS) Office on Minority Health (OWH) Minority Women's Health Panel of Experts, served on the U.S. DHHS–Centers for Medicare & Medicaid Services' Advisory Panel on Outreach and Education, and the U.S. DHHS–OWH Region IX Women's Health Advisory Council, cochaired the International Association of Gerontology and Geriatrics 2017 World Congress on Gerontology and Geriatrics Local Arrangements Committee and the Regional Health Equity Council for Region IX (RHEC IX).

Dr. Yee-Melichar is a charter Fellow of the Academy for Gerontology in Higher Education; Fellow of the Gerontological Society of America; Fellow of the American Alliance for Health, Physical Education, Recreation and Dance Research Consortium; and member of Sigma Xi, the National Research Society. She has served on the editorial boards of the Journal of Gerontological Social Work, Journal of Health Education, and other peer-reviewed publications. She also serves on the board of directors for the California Advocates for Nursing Home Reform (CANHR), as an OMH Health Equity Mentor for the U.S. DHHS, and on the Cal MediConnect (CMC) Advisory Committee of the San Mateo Health Commission.

She received her BA in biology from Barnard College, MS in gerontology from the College of New Rochelle, and MS and EdD in health education focusing on gerontology from Columbia University.

Cristina Flores, PhD, RN, FGSA, has been a registered nurse for more than 30 years. Her nursing practice has included many aspects of the continuum of care, such as home health care, assisted living communities, and the acute care hospital. She holds an MA in gerontology from San Francisco State University (SF State) and a PhD in nursing health policy from the University of California, San Francisco (UCSF). She is the former owner and licensee of three six-bed residential care facilities for the elderly in California, a lecturer in the gerontology program at SF State, and an adjunct professor for UCSF. She has published several journal articles, book chapters, and three books relative to long-term care administration and quality of care. She is a Fellow of the Gerontological Society of America, a member of the Governing Board of the National Consumer Voice for Quality Long-Term Care, and was the recipient of the 2009 Kenji Murase Distinguished Alumni Award, School of Social Work, SF State.

Andrea Renwanz Boyle, PhD, RN, FNAP, is a graduate of the University of California, San Francisco, where she received a PhD in nursing science. Dr. Boyle received her MS in nursing from Boston University and adult nurse practitioner certification from Peter Bent Brigham Hospital. Currently, Dr. Boyle is the associate dean and professor of nursing at Dominican University of California and a Distinguished Practice Fellow in the National Academies of Practice. Dr. Boyle is the President of Sigma Theta Tau International Nursing Honor Society (Rho Alpha Chapter) and an emerita associate professor at San Francisco State University. Dr. Boyle is widely published in the areas of health-related issues in aging and assisted living, nursing education, evidence-based practice, problem-based learning, and interprofessional practice in palliative care. She has presented her work at a number of international and national scholarly research and professional conferences and currently serves as a manuscript reviewer for interprofessional, geriatric, and nursing journals. Dr. Boyle has served as a member of national and international nursing boards and organizations, including the International Council of Nurses Nurse Practitioner/Advanced Practice Nursing Network and the Regional Health Equity Council for Region IX (RHEC IX). Dr. Boyle has served as a commissioner on the California Workforce Policy Commission, been certified as a residential care facility for the elderly (RCFE) administrator, and worked in primary care settings as an adult and geriatric nurse practitioner. Dr. Boyle received the 2009 SF State Distinguished Faculty Award for Excellence in Service.

ASSISTED LIVING ADMINISTRATION AND MANAGEMENT REVIEW

Practice Questions for RC/AL Administrator Certification/Licensure

Darlene Yee-Melichar, EdD, FGSA, FAGHE

Cristina Flores, PhD, RN, FGSA

Andrea Renwanz Boyle, PhD, RN, FNAP

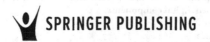 SPRINGER PUBLISHING

Springer Publishing Company, LLC
11 West 42nd Street, New York, NY 10036
www.springerpub.com
connect.springerpub.com/

Acquisitions Editor: David D'Addona
Compositor: S4Carlisle Publishing Services

ISBN: 978-0-8261-6734-7
ebook ISBN: 978-0-8261-6735-4
DOI: 10.1891/9780826167354

21 22 23 24 / 5 4 3 2 1

Library of Congress Cataloging-in-Publication Data

Names: Yee-Melichar, Darlene, author. | Flores, Cristina M., author. |
  Boyle, Andrea Renwanz, author.
Title: Assisted living administration and management review : practice
  questions for RC/AL administrator certification/licensure / Darlene
  Yee-Melichar, EdD, FGSA, FAGHE, Cristina Flores, PhD, RN, FGSA, Andrea
  Renwanz Boyle, PhD, RN, FNAP.
Description: New York : Springer Publishing, [2022] | Includes
  bibliographical references and index.
Identifiers: LCCN 2021047098 (print) | LCCN 2021047099 (ebook) | ISBN
  9780826167347 (cloth) | ISBN 9780826167354 (ebook)
Subjects: LCSH: Congregate housing--Management. | Old age homes. | Nursing
  homes.
Classification: LCC HV1454 .Y45 2022 (print) | LCC HV1454 (ebook) | DDC
  362.61--dc23/eng/20211109
LC record available at https://lccn.loc.gov/2021047098
LC ebook record available at https://lccn.loc.gov/2021047099
LCCN: 2021047098

Contact sales@springerpub.com to receive discount rates on bulk purchases.

Publisher's Note: New and used products purchased from third-party sellers are not guaranteed for quality, authenticity, or access to any included digital components.

Printed in the United States of America.

Dedicated to the students and practitioners in health and human services who are committed to enhancing the quality of care and quality of life of older adults residing in assisted living facilities and other long-term care communities.

With love and gratitude to our families and friends for their continuing patience and moral support

CONTENTS

CONTRIBUTORS

Victoria Aguila, MA, Housekeeping Manager, Channing House, Palo Alto, California

Yadira Aldana, MA, Director of Operations, Channing House, Palo Alto, California

Mark Cimino, JD, CEO, CiminoCare, Sacramento, California

Mia Enriquez, MA, Owner, Tara Hills Care Home/DMC Homes Inc., Pinole, California

Terry Ervin, MBA, Executive Director, Oakmont Senior Living, Sacramento, California

Pauline Mosher Shatara, MA, Deputy Director, California Advocates for Nursing Home Reform, Berkeley, California

Ismael Tellez, MA, Project Policy Analyst, University of California San Francisco PREPARE Program, San Francisco, California

Connie Yuen, MA, Executive Director, St. Paul's Towers, Oakland, California

ACKNOWLEDGMENTS

We are grateful to the many people who have contributed meaningfully to the successful completion of *Assisted Living Administration and Management Review: Practice Questions for RC/AL Administrator Certification/Licensure* (also known as this *Review Book*).

In particular, we thank David D'Addona and Jaclyn Shultz at Springer Publishing Company, who helped to enhance and extend *Assisted Living Administration and Management: Effective Practices and Model Programs in Elder Care (Second Edition)* with this *Review Book*. We appreciated very much the encouragement, patience, and support that our colleagues at Springer Publishing have provided during the past year in broadening and enriching our efforts on an important area of study.

We especially wish to thank the contributing authors who have shared their respective areas of expertise with us in this *Review Book*. Victoria Aguila, MA; Yadira Aldana, MA; Mark J. Cimino, JD; Mia Enriquez, MA; Terry Ervin, MBA; Pauline Mosher Shatara, MA; Ismael Tellez, MA; and Connie Yuen, MA, are to be commended for contributing to the thoughtful questions and answers provided. Their informed, insightful, and invaluable contributions are an asset to the *Review Book*. Thank you all for the successful teamwork.

San Francisco State University student assistants Rayeil Laia and Sina Riahi provided helpful assistance with detailing rationales and updating references. Your behind-the-scenes support was much appreciated.

Our families and friends have been a mainstay of encouragement and support throughout the preparation of this *Review Book*, and we take this opportunity to express our gratitude to all of them:

- Joseph and Helen Melichar, and Yuen Hing and Raymond Yee
- Robert and Irene Benjamin, Jacqueline and Jake Angelo, and Albert Ujcic
- Robert and Bubba Boyle

We could not have done this without you—thank you all for your help and support in making this *Review Book* the best it could be.

INTRODUCTION

POPULATION AGING IS ON THE RISE

An aging population is one in which the number and proportion of older people increases over time. This is referred to as demographic aging or population aging. Demographic changes since the second half of the last century have led to a global aging population, resulting in important economic and social concerns worldwide. The main causes of aging populations are declining fertility rates and increasing life expectancy (United Nations, Department of Economic and Social Affairs, Population Division, 2019).

This transformation caused by a rapidly aging population in the United States has been referred to as "the graying of America" or "the silver tsunami." Notably, in the United States and throughout the rest of the world, the "Baby Boomer" generation began to turn 65 in 2011. Recently, the population aged 65 years and older has grown at a faster rate than the total population in the United States (U.S. Census Bureau, 2020).

The total population increased by 9.7%, from 281.4 million to 308.7 million, between 2000 and 2010. Yet, the population aged 65 years and older increased by 15.1% during the same period. It has been estimated that 25% of the population in the United States and Canada will be aged 65 years and older by 2025. Moreover, by 2050, it is predicted that, for the first time in U.S. history, the number of individuals aged 60 years and older will be greater than the number of children aged 0 to 14 years (Target Health, 2017).

Those aged 85 years and older (oldest-old) are projected to increase from 5.3 million to 21 million by 2050. Adults aged 85 to 89 years constituted the greatest segment of the oldest-old in 1990, 2000, and 2010. However, the largest percentage point increase among the oldest-old occurred in the 90- to 94-year-old age group, which increased from 25.0% in 1990 to 26.4% in 2010. It is especially important to note that "aging in America" is becoming more diverse (U.S. Census Bureau, 2011a).

There has been a disparity between the number of men and women in the older population in the United States. Although the gender gap between men and women has narrowed, women continue to have a greater life expectancy and lower mortality rates at older ages relative to men. For example, the Census 2010 reported that there were approximately twice as many women as men living in the United States at 89 years of age (361,309 vs. 176,689, respectively). In 2018, older women outnumbered older men at 29.1 million older women to 23.3 million older men (U.S. Census Bureau, 2011b).

In 2018, 23% of persons age 65 and older were members of racial or ethnic minority populations: 9% were African Americans (not Hispanic), 5% were Asian (not Hispanic), 0.5% were American Indian and Alaska Native (not Hispanic), 0.1% were Native Hawaiian/Pacific Islander (not Hispanic), and 0.8% of persons 65 and older identified themselves as being of two or more races. Persons of Hispanic origin (who may be of any race) represented 8% of the older population (Administration on Aging, 2020). It is clear that both the aging and diversity of the population need much more attention in the United States.

The U.S. Census Bureau (2020) released 2019 population estimates by demographic characteristics. In Figure 1, three census infographics are available that present:

1. a wave of change: age structure of the U.S. resident population by sex,

2. older and growing: percent change among the 65 and older population, and

3. the next generation: percent change among the under 18 population.

Several states (California, Colorado, Massachusetts, Minnesota, and Texas) have taken the lead in creating Master Plans for Aging to address the needs of diverse, older adults for long-term

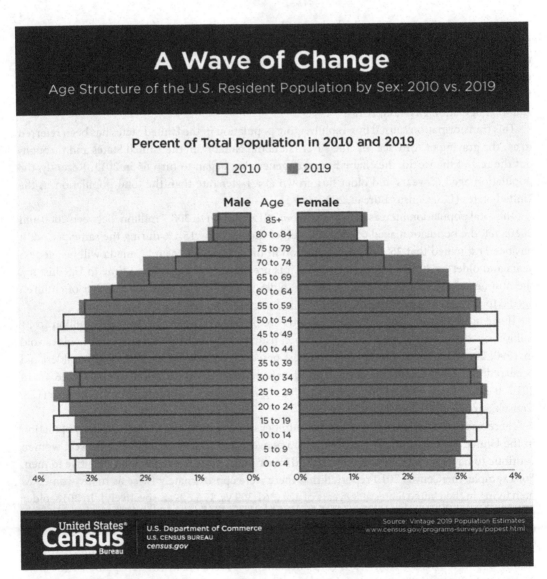

FIGURE 1 U.S. Census Bureau infographics.

Source: U.S. Census Bureau. (2020, June). *65 and older population grows rapidly as Baby Boomers age* [Press release]. https://www.census.gov/newsroom/press-releases/2020/65-older-population-grows.html

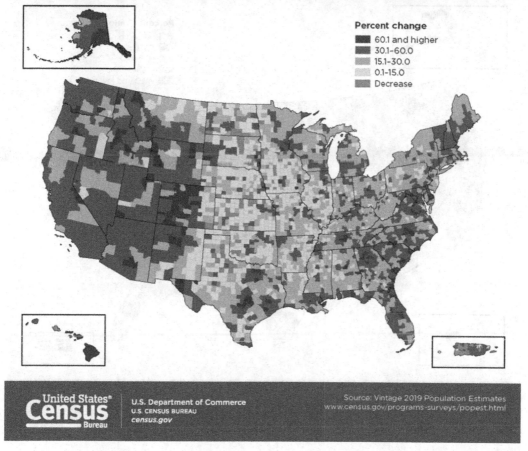

Older and Growing
Percent Change among the 65 and Older Population: 2010 to 2019

Percent change
- 60.1 and higher
- 30.1–60.0
- 15.1–30.0
- 0.1–15.0
- Decrease

United States Census Bureau
U.S. Department of Commerce
U.S. CENSUS BUREAU
census.gov

Source: Vintage 2019 Population Estimates
www.census.gov/programs-surveys/popest.html

FIGURE 1 (continued)

services and supports (LTSS). For example, recognizing that California's over-65 population is projected to grow to 8.6 million by 2030, Governor Gavin Newsom issued an executive order calling for the creation of a Master Plan for Aging.

The Master Plan will serve as a blueprint that can be used by state government, local communities, private organizations, and philanthropy to build environments that promote an age friendly California. This innovative Master Plan for Aging in California was released on January 6, 2021 (https://www.chhs.ca.gov/home/master-plan-for-aging/). Box 1 outlines five bold goals and targets to build a California for All Ages by 2030. It also includes a Data Dashboard for Aging to measure progress and a Local Playbook to drive partnerships that help meet these goals.

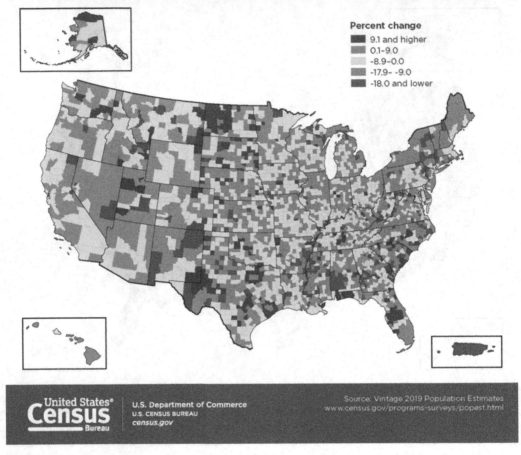

The Next Generation

Percent Change among the Under 18 Population: 2010 to 2019

Percent change
- 9.1 and higher
- 0.1–9.0
- -8.9–0.0
- -17.9– -9.0
- -18.0 and lower

United States® Census Bureau
U.S. Department of Commerce
U.S. CENSUS BUREAU
census.gov

Source: Vintage 2019 Population Estimates
www.census.gov/programs-surveys/popest.html

FIGURE 1 *(continued)*

BOX 1   CALIFORNIA'S MASTER PLAN FOR AGING'S FIVE BOLD GOALS FOR 2030.

■ **Goal One: Housing for All Ages and Stages**
   ■ We will live where we choose as we age in communities that are age-, disability-, and dementia-friendly and climate- and disaster-ready.
   ■ Target: Millions of New Housing Options to Age Well

■ **Goal Two: Health Reimagined**
   ■ We will have access to the services we need to live at home in our communities and to optimize our health and quality of life.
   ■ Target: Close the Equity Gap in and Increase Life Expectancy

(continued)

GERONTOLOGY EDUCATION AND TRAINING ESSENTIAL

With the rapid growth of the aging population, the demand for gerontology education and training for those interested in older adults and practitioners interested in working with older adults are increasingly in demand. Gerontology is the study of aging processes and individuals across the life course. Gerontology includes the study of biomedical, psychosocial, and socioeconomic changes in people as they age; the scientific research of changes in society resulting from our aging population; and the application of this new knowledge to innovative policies and programs.

Gerontology is distinguished from geriatrics, which is the branch of medicine that specializes in the prevention and treatment of existing disease in older adults. Gerontology is multidisciplinary in that it combines and/or integrates several different areas of study. Gerontologists include educators, researchers and practitioners in various fields such as biology, business, counseling, dentistry, economics, housing, kinesiology, medicine, nursing, occupational therapy, pharmacy, physical therapy, political science, psychology, psychiatry, public administration, public health, social work, sociology, and more.

As a result of the multidisciplinary focus of gerontology, professionals from diverse fields call themselves gerontologists. Gerontologists help to improve the quality of care, quality of life and promote the well-being of people as they age through research, education, practice, and the application of interdisciplinary knowledge of the aging process and aging populations. The multidisciplinary nature of gerontology means that there are a number of subfields that overlap with gerontology.

For instance, there are policy issues involved in government planning and the operation of skilled nursing facilities (SNF), investigating the effects of an aging population on society, and the design of residential spaces for older people that facilitate the development of a sense of place or home. Dr. M. Powell Lawton, a behavioral psychologist at the at the Weiss Pavilion at the Philadelphia Geriatric Center, was among the first to recognize the need for living spaces designed to accommodate older adults, especially those with Alzheimer's disease and related disorders. With a preventative focus on aging in community, the AARP Network of Age-Friendly States and Communities was established in April 2012 as an independent affiliate of the World Health Organization (WHO) Global Network for Age-Friendly Cities and Communities (www .aarp.org/livable-communities/network-age-friendly-communities/).

As an academic discipline, gerontology is relatively new. An *Online Directory of Educational Programs in Gerontology* is available at www.aghedirectory.org/. The Online Directory was made possible through a grant from Archstone Foundation to the Academy for Gerontology in Higher Education (AGHE). This online tool is an easy-to-use resource that allows you to browse educational programs by location, type of degree program, certificate, or fellowship offered.

Exemplars include a private university, the University of Southern California Leonard Davis School, which created the first doctoral, master's, and bachelor's degree programs in gerontology in 1975. As part of public higher education in the California State University (CSU) system, San Francisco State University (SF State) created the first Master of Arts (MA) degree program in gerontology in 1986. SF State's MA degree in gerontology prepares students for effectively serving the needs of diverse groups of older adults. It also lays a firm academic foundation in applied gerontology for those who choose to work toward a doctoral or professional degree.

Like other gerontology education programs of merit, SF State's graduate gerontology program is dedicated to (a) interdisciplinary education, (b) multiple approaches to meeting the needs of the diverse aging population, (c) research to expand bodies of knowledge about aging, (d) effective practice relevant to aging populations, and (e) community applications to advocate for improving the quality of life for older individuals. Students may choose a number of career paths in the field of aging within the public and private sectors.

CAREERS IN AGING ARE SIGNIFICANT

The Gerontological Society of America (GSA) hosts a website to assist individuals with their professional career in the field of gerontology. *AgeWork* (https://agework.geron.org/) helps connect talent with opportunity. Job seekers can find their employment of choice and employers can reach the most qualified candidates in the field of aging. Other GSA career resources (www.geron.org/career-center) include (a) videos and vignettes, (b) online resources, and (c) tip sheets.

Videos and vignettes include, but are not limited to, The Real Faces of Careers in Aging, Academic Job Market: What Every Early Professional Needs to Know, Non-Academic Careers in Aging; Trends in Aging, and More Than Just Memes: Using Social Media and Technology to Boost Your Career. Online resources include, but are not limited to, Exploring Careers in Aging: A Roadmap for Students, American Health Care Association/National Center for Assisted Living (AHCA/NCAL) Workforce Resource Center, LeadingAge Center for Workforce Solutions, and Senior Living Works. Tip sheets include, but are not limited to, Challenges and Solutions in Mentoring Relationships, Developing and Maintaining a Professional Identity, How to Balance Work and Family Life, Interviewing Strategies 101, and Seven Tips for Successfully Negotiating a Job Offer.

It is apparent that the assisted living/residential care profession is on a trajectory for significant job growth. For example, the online site for the AHCA/NCAL Workforce Resource Center (www.ahcancal.org/Workforce-and-Career/Pages/Organizations.aspx) includes numerous resources for long-term care (LTC) organizations. These include, but are not limited to,

(a) LTC Career Center (www.ahcancal.org/Workforce-and-Career/Pages/LTC-Career-Center.aspx) seeking high-quality, professional individuals to be a part of the team. LTC organizations can post jobs online quickly and easily manage applications, search resumes, and set up alerts, and (b) ConnectToCareJobs (www.connecttocarejobs.com/#/) is a free national website that provides an easy way for LTC employers to connect with individuals looking for jobs. The tool uses a matching algorithm to pair licensed and/or trained workers with healthcare facilities that are in need of their specific skills.

The California Assisted Living Association (CALA, an Argentum State Partner) website has an informative section on workforce development (https://caassistedliving.org/workforce/) with tools and resources to help Assisted Living, Memory Care, and CCRC (continuing care retirement community) practitioners develop and sustain a workforce ready to meet these escalating needs. Whether through community partners serving as guest lecturers, internship preceptors, and/or participating in a careers-in-aging job fair, building relationships by offering student-learning opportunities can help develop the much-needed workforce in assisted living/residential care communities.

Students interested in learning more about the assisted living/residential care profession can apply for scholarship support, through organizations like CALA, to attend a professional conference. Participation at a professional conference will enable students to (a) gain a greater understanding of the assisted living/residential care profession, (b) meet face-to-face with prospective employers online or on-site at the professional conference, (c) attend cutting-edge educational sessions and network with assisted living/residential care professionals, and (d) hear from an assisted living/residential care professional who could share strategies to navigating a career path. Furthermore, from the assisted living/residential care professional perspective, research shows building a team of quality student interns—who are then employed as staff members—leads to a high quality of life for residents.

The LeadingAge Center for Workforce Solutions (https://leadingage.org/workforce) features workforce resources for older adult services. LTC practitioners and students will find an info graphic on the National Workforce Crisis facing LTSS (https://leadingage.org/sites/default/files/LA_Workforce_Infographics_FULLPAGE%202%2020.pdf) as well as promising practices for recruitment, retention, and collaborations; recruitment tools; workforce tools; and other information and strategies that will help build a quality workforce.

Careers in aging leading to more quality residential care/assisted living administrators are significant in meeting the needs of older adults. According to the Centers for Disease Control and Prevention (CDC; www.cdc.gov/nchs/fastats/residential-care-communities.htm), there are 28,900 residential care communities with 996,100 licensed beds and 811,500 residents in the United States.

PROFESSIONAL CREDENTIALS ARE IMPERATIVE

According to Professional Testing, Inc. (2006, pp. 1–2), certification and licensure tests have a number of elements in common, along with a few important differences. Both types of tests are criterion-referenced tests, and both are used to measure the knowledge and skills related to particular jobs. While the terms are not used with complete consistency, the term *certification* most often refers to a voluntary exam program sponsored by an agency related to the occupation, for the purpose of measuring professional competency. In contrast, the term *licensure* usually refers to a government-sponsored program that an individual is legally required to complete, before they can be employed in the occupation. The two types of tests may also differ in terms of their overall test purposes and in the additional requirements the sponsoring agency may have for the candidates.

Certification and licensure programs typically have different primary test purposes. Certification tests are often designed to measure a broad set of knowledge and skills that an individual working in a particular occupation ought to have. In many instances, a professional organization has developed a set of standards for professional practice, and the certification exam is designed to measure these standards. While certification tests may be designed to measure entry-level skills, or minimal competency, they may also be aimed at a specialty level or an advanced level of professional practice. In licensure programs, on the other hand, the focus of the test is directly on protecting health, safety, and welfare. Licensure tests are usually aimed at protecting public safety by ensuring a minimum degree of competency on the part of the candidates.

Perhaps the most obvious difference between certification and licensure programs is whether they are elective or mandatory for the examinees. Certification tests are programs designed for the purpose of measuring professional competency; they may be sponsored by associations, corporations, or academic institutions. While certification tests are legally voluntary, passing such an exam is sometimes required by an employer before an individual can be hired or promoted. Government-sponsored licensure tests, on the other hand, are typically legally mandatory for any individual who wishes to be employed in the job or profession.

Both certification and licensure programs often have specific eligibility requirements for the candidate, and they are both usually granted for a specific, limited period. In addition, both types of programs often have ongoing requirements for the individual to maintain the certification or license. These ongoing requirements might include continuing education and/or retesting.

While both certification and licensure tests are designed to measure examinee competence in some job-related area, there are important distinctions. These include whether the primary purpose of the test is concerned with professional competence or public safety and whether the exam is voluntary or mandatory for the examinee.

RESIDENTIAL CARE/ASSISTED LIVING ADMINISTRATOR CERTIFICATION/LICENSURE

In addition to academic credentials in gerontology education and training, state certification/licensure in residential care/assisted living administration is strongly recommended. Unlike the Nursing Home Administrator licensure exam, there is *no federal requirement* for residential care/assisted living administrator certification/licensure at this time. Each state sets its own residential care/assisted living regulations and administers its own certification/licensure examination. The NCAL publishes the *Assisted Living State Regulatory Review* on an annual basis; it is a comprehensive report where you can check the most current regulations for your state (www.ahcancal.org/Assisted-Living/Policy/Documents/2019_reg_review.pdf).

According to Dr. James E. Allen (2004), the National Association of Boards of Examiners for Long-Term Care Administrators (NAB) initiated a job analysis of the practice of assisted living administration in 1996. In 1997, the NAB recommended five areas in which the assisted living administrator should be knowledgeable: (a) organizational management, (b) human resources management, (c) business/financial management, (d) physical environment management, and (e) resident care management. In 1998, the NAB began offering an *elective* national examination covering these five knowledge areas or domains of practice for those wishing to become professional assisted living administrators.

The National Association of Long-Term Care Administrator Boards (NAB) states that it conducts a Professional Practice Analysis (PPA) every 5 years to ensure that its licensure exams accurately represent the current scope of practice of the profession. The new PPA serves as the

TABLE 1 NAB'S NEW DOMAINS OF PRACTICE—2022

CURRENT DOMAINS, EFFECTIVE 2017	NEW DOMAINS, EFFECTIVE IN MARCH 2022
10. Customer Care, Supports, and Services	1. Care, Services, and Supports
20. Human Resource	2. Operations
30. Finance	
40. Environment	3. Environmental and Quality
50. Management and Leadership	4. Leadership and Strategy

Source: NAB. (n.d.) *New domains of practice—2022*. https://www.nabweb.org/nab-domains-of-practice-2

foundation for the exams, as well as content for continuing education, academic programs, exam prep study material, and standards of practice for state licensing boards. While most of the knowledge and tasks have not changed significantly, they have been realigned from five to four domains of practice effective in 2022 (https://www.nabweb.org/nab-domains-of-practice-2; Table 1).

In addition, an *elective* Certified Director of Assisted Living (CDAL) program may be used as a means of promoting professionalism within the senior living industry. The CDAL program is administered under the authority of the Senior Living Certification Commission (SLCC), which is part of Argentum. Argentum is the leading national trade association serving companies that own, operate, and support professionally managed senior living communities in the United States (www.argentum.org/assisted-living-executive-director-certification-program/).

Ongoing and continuing education for residential care/assisted living administrators and their interprofessional team members remains a cornerstone for excellence in elder care delivery. Mandated trainings, professional continuing education, specialty care training, and disaster management trainings addressing natural disasters and the recent COVID-19 pandemic represent educational areas of importance for administrators, practitioners, staff, and residents.

Assisted living administrators are required to stay current with state-mandated regulations and national recommendations and guidelines. Education for assisted living administrators and interprofessional team members includes state-mandated core trainings and program trainings focused on the domains of practice. These domains of practice include organizational management, human resource management, business and financial management, environmental management, and resident care management. Requirements for mandated institutional trainings in each state are described in reviews of assisted living regulations (National Center for Assisted Living, 2019) and should be a major component of required educational programs.

Practitioners working in assisted living/residential care communities update their understanding of elder care delivery for residents through a number of formal professional continuing education programs. Updated information in content on physical aspects of aging, such as memory care, nutrition, medication administration, and management of illnesses, including heart disease and strokes, are examples of areas where professionals regularly improve their education. Continuing education programs are offered through professional organizations, universities, state licensing boards, and private companies. One example of a state level organization is the Florida Senior Living Association (FSLA), whose annual conferences, continuing education courses, and certification exam review questions enable assisted living administrators, practitioners, and staff to remain current through broad-based educational offerings (https://floridaseniorliving.org/).

Assisted living community members must remain current in understanding and management of emergencies and disasters. The COVID-19 pandemic presents a new and growing national challenge for administrators, practitioners, staff, and residents as well as for family and friends of assisted living residents. Members of assisted living communities, especially residents and staff members from at-risk demographic groups, remain at significant risk for morbidity and mortality associated with COVID-19. Current and ongoing education is critical for providing administrators and practitioners with effective practices to keep vulnerable assisted living community members safe through the diagnosis, assessment, and management of COVID-19 by offering coronavirus testing, contact tracing, quarantine, and current medical treatments. Federal and state guidelines from the Centers of Disease Control and Prevention, the U.S. Public Health Department, state and local public health departments, and medical and elder organization trainings are examples of educational efforts to provide necessary information during the current healthcare crisis.

DOMAINS OF PRACTICE AND AREAS OF RESPONSIBILITY FOR RESIDENTIAL CARE/ASSISTED LIVING CERTIFICATION/LICENSURE EXAMINATION

For the purposes of this *Review Book*, the five knowledge areas or domains of practice identified by the NAB in 1997 were further explored in relation to available state mandates (e.g., California Code of Regulations, Title 22, Division 6, Chapter 8, Section 87405; https://govt.westlaw.com/calregs/Document/IDB071D9E4B644F60A7051A439F2C2BD3?viewType=FullText&originationContext=documenttoc&transitionType=CategoryPageItem&contextData=(sc.Default)&bhcp=1) for residential care/assisted living administrators.

The five domains of practice in this *Review Book* can be compared and contrasted to the four domains identified in the NAB criteria effective 2022 (www.nabweb.org/nab-domains-of-practice-2). Except for the NAB's realignment from five to four domains of practice, the content information, knowledge base, and tasks are equivalent.

Each of the five parts of this *Review Book* focuses sequentially on the five domains of practice resulting from this comparative analysis. It is evident that this *Review Book* has retained the initial knowledge areas or domains of practice; the *Review Book* also reflects the Second Edition of *Assisted Living Administration and Management: Effective Practices and Model Programs in Elder Care* (Yee-Melichar et al., 2021) upon which it is based. Part One covers Domain of Practice 1, organizational management; Part Two explores Domain of Practice 2, human resources management; Part Three focuses on Domain of Practice 3, business and financial management; Part Four includes Domain of Practice 4, Environmental management; and Part Five involves Domain of Practice 5, Resident care management (Table 2).

TABLE 2 *SECOND EDITION* AND *REVIEW BOOK* DOMAINS OF PRACTICE AND CONTENT AREAS FOR RESIDENTIAL CARE/ASSISTED LIVING ADMINISTRATION KNOWLEDGE BASE

DOMAINS OF PRACTICE	CONTENT AREAS FOR KNOWLEDGE BASE
1, Organizational Management	The Assisted Living Industry: Context, History, Overview
	Policy, Licensing, and Regulations
	Organizational Overview
2, Human Resources Management	Recruiting and Hiring Staff
	Training Staff
	Retaining Employees with Empowerment

(continued)

TABLE 2 *SECOND EDITION* AND *REVIEW BOOK* DOMAINS OF PRACTICE AND CONTENT AREAS FOR RESIDENTIAL CARE/ASSISTED LIVING ADMINISTRATION KNOWLEDGE BASE

	Continuing Education
	Interprofessional Practice: Issues for Assisted Living Administrators
3, Business and Financial Management	Business, Management, and Marketing
	Financial Management in Assisted Living Communities
	Legal Concepts and Issues in Assisted Living Communities
4, Environmental Management	Accessibility, Fire Safety, and Disaster Preparedness
	Models of Care
	Universal Design and Aging in Place
	Home- and Community-Based Services as an Alternative to Assisted Living
	Information and Communication Technology in Assisted Living
5, Resident Care Management	Diversity Issues
	LGBTQ Issues in Assisted Living
	Physical Aspects of Aging
	Psychological Aspects of Aging
	Memory Care in Assisted Living: Benefits and Challenges for Administrators
	Palliative and Hospice Care
	Residents' Rights

Source: Yee-Melichar, D., Flores, C., & Boyle, A. R. (2021). *Assisted living administration and management: Effective practices and model programs in elder care* (2nd ed.). Springer. https://www.springerpub.com/assisted-living-administration-and-management-9780826161949.html

PART ONE: ORGANIZATIONAL MANAGEMENT

This domain covers three main areas that are essential to the knowledge base of the assisted living administrator: (1) The Assisted Living Industry: Context, History, and Overview; (2) Policy, Licensing, and Regulations; and (3) Organizational Overview.

Area 1 focuses on the basic concepts of assisted living, including historical background, nomenclature, definitions, and a description of the industry. The evolution and emergence of assisted living is considered. Operational definitions of industry-specific terms are included. Furthermore, common resident characteristics (e.g., demographics) are identified. Assisted living administrators need to be familiar with these fundamental concepts as a basis for understanding their role and responsibilities.

Area 2 focuses on laws and regulations regarding assisted living and the similarities and differences across states. Generically describing assisted living policy, licensing, and regulations is challenging as states are individually responsible for the oversight of assisted living. Administrators will need to identify and become familiar with their own states' (a) regulatory agency, (b) applicable laws and regulations, (c) policies and procedures, and (d) funding streams for reimbursement. The administrator must also understand federal laws and statutes that may apply to their communities (e.g., Americans with Disabilities Act).

Area 3 provides an overview of the organizational patterns and models used in the assisted living industry. Understanding the concept of "aging in place" in the context of assisted living is essential. The administrator must have knowledge of the variety in patterns and models as they are affected by many factors, including size and type of service model. This area highlights the need for today's assisted living administrators to be well informed and remain attuned to the evolving needs, practices, and models in the industry.

PART TWO: HUMAN RESOURCES MANAGEMENT

This domain covers five main areas that are essential to the knowledge base of the assisted living administrator: (1) Recruiting and Hiring Staff, (2) Training Staff, (3) Retaining Employees with Empowerment, (4) Continuing Education, and (5) Interprofessional Practice: Issues for Assisted Living Administrators.

Area 1 provides an understanding of why the success of an assisted living community depends greatly on the hiring of appropriate staff that is based on the specific needs of the community. It describes the recruitment and hiring of suitable staff persons, including the administrator and direct care workers. Factors influencing recruitment, recruitment sources, and hiring process are stressed to illustrate their importance.

Area 2 includes the training processes of staff in assisted living. Concepts such as orientation, on-the-job training, and the evaluation of training processes are incorporated. The administrator should identify their own state's specific laws and requirements for training.

Area 3 illustrates strategies for the retention of key and high-quality personnel. The needs of employees, such as economic security and job satisfaction, are considered. Strategies for empowering staff to participate in the vision of the assisted living community are highlighted.

Area 4 emphasizes staff development concepts, including continuing education requirements for personnel. An overview of the various state requirements for ongoing training and continuing education for the administrator and direct care staff is included. The administrator must identify their own state's specific laws and requirements for continuing education.

Area 5 describes the important need for interprofessional practice roles in assisted living communities. Definitions of *interprofessional practice*, descriptions of interprofessional team member roles, and benefits and issues of interprofessional practice are included.

PART THREE: BUSINESS AND FINANCIAL MANAGEMENT

This domain covers three main areas that are essential to the knowledge base of the assisted living administrator: (1) Business, Management, and Marketing; (2) Financial Management in Assisted Living Communities; and (3) Legal Concepts and Issues in Assisted Living Communities.

Area 1 provides an understanding of business, management, and marketing concepts in assisted living communities with attention to management theories and how they can be implemented; management method and style important to assisted living community operations, planning framework for efficient and effective assisted living community management and organizational structure, business and operational plans, information and technology support systems, and marketing approaches for assisted living communities.

Area 2 includes financial information on accounting systems, organization, financial reporting, account procedures, accounts records, budget preparation, ratio analysis, risk management, and accounting terms used in assisted living communities. This area also includes information about generally accepted accounting principles; National Investment Center for Senior Housing; real estate aspects of assisted living communities, such as lease agreements and real estate investment trusts (REITs); differences between a publicly traded company versus privately held versus nonprofits (charity and noncharities) and the reporting obligations associated; and financial analysis using proformas for acquisitions or ground-up start-ups.

Area 3 describes fundamental legal information on tort law and negligence, respondeat superior, corporate negligence, governing body, contracts, evictions, wills, trusts, conservatorships, guardianships, advance directives, living wills, and durable power of attorney.

PART FOUR: ENVIRONMENTAL MANAGEMENT

This domain covers five main areas that are essential to the knowledge base of the assisted living administrator: (1) Accessibility, Fire Safety, and Disaster Preparedness; (2) Models of Care; (3) Universal Design and Aging in Place; (4) Home and Community-Based Service Alternatives to Assisted Living; and (5) Information and Communication Technology.

Area 1 provides the assisted living administrator with a brief review of selected federal regulations, laws, and statutes related to disaster preparedness and accessibility as well as information about National Fire Protection Associations. Major issues related to accessibility, fire safety, and disaster preparedness are identified as critical as are strategies for fire and disaster preparedness. Assisted living administrators are provided with information on disaster preparations, disaster protection, and recovery from disasters as well as selected resources to address disasters.

Area 2 provides information on methods of service delivery in assisted living communities. Descriptions of culture change and care delivery models, including the medical model, Greenhouse model, and Eden Alternative, can help administrators consider options and best practices for eldercare delivery in assisted living settings. Enhanced understanding of some of the benefits and challenges associated with each of the identified care models can also be valuable for administrators.

Area 3 is focused on universal design and aging in place. Administrators can benefit from understanding definitions, philosophy, and key principles of universal design as well as strategies to connect these concepts to the structure of assisted living communities. Administrators and staff members can help assisted living residents and family members through the use of aging-in-place strategies including space and product design.

Area 4 is designed to provide assisted living administrators with information about home and community-based services (HCBS) as components of LTC and assisted living services. Awareness of the history and the structure of three HCBS programs including State Plan, 1915c, and PACE allows for possible expansion of HCBS in light of current consumer challenges.

Area 5 includes an introduction and descriptions of information and communication technology (ICT). The use of ICT offers both benefits and challenges to assisted living administrators, staff, and residents. Additionally, ICT can be viewed as a tool for safeguarding residents who are aging in place while overall resident quality-of-life enhancements.

PART FIVE: RESIDENT CARE MANAGEMENT

This domain covers seven main areas that are essential to the knowledge base of the assisted living administrator: (1) Diversity Issues, (2) Lesbian-Gay-Bisexual-Transgender (LGBT) Issues in Assisted Living, (3) Physical Aspects of Aging, (4) Psychological Aspects of Aging, (5) Memory Care Units in Assisted Living: Benefits and Challenges for Administrators, (6) Palliative and Hospice Care, and (7) Residents' Rights.

Area 1 provides the assisted living administrator with the information needed to understand and work with staff and residents from diverse cultural and social groups. An understanding of these differences aids in the administrator's success. African Americans, Hispanics, Asian Americans, and Native Americans are highlighted as groups with diverse needs.

Area 2 addresses the urgent need to acknowledge and learn about the unique fundamentals of LGBT older adults. The historical context and critical issues need to be understood by the assisted living administrator. The administrator must develop their skills to address the challenges and barriers faced by LGBT residents.

Area 3 aids the assisted living administrator by providing knowledge of physiologic changes that normally occur in the body systems as people age. These include changes to the cardiovascular, respiratory, muscular, orthopedic, gastrointestinal, genitourinary, skin, lymphatic, and neurological systems. An understanding of these changes allows the administrator to identify and address problems resulting from normal age-related physical changes. Commonly occurring issues such as nutrition, mobility, fall prevention, sleep, and chronic pain management are emphasized.

Area 4 considers the normal aging-related changes in neurological functioning, mental health functioning, memory, and cognition and their effects on the psychological well-being of residents. By understanding these changes, the administrator can have an awareness of the needs of residents and develop appropriate interventions to address them.

Area 5 addresses the ever-changing and developing need for memory care. With the numbers of elders dealing with neurocognitive disorder (formerly known as dementia) expected to increase on a global level within the next 20 years, so will the need for memory care services. The assisted living administrator needs to understand the benefits and challenges associated with the elements and management of memory care units.

Area 6 focuses on palliative and hospice care, also an area of rapid growth and change within the assisted living industry. Residents with life-threatening illnesses or critically progressed from their chronic diseases can benefit greatly from appropriate palliative and hospice programs. In an effort to allow residents to remain in their assisted living community as their needs change, the administrator must understand the philosophies and modalities of palliative care and hospice care. Additionally, the administrator should understand any associated laws and regulations.

Area 7 concentrates on the rights of residents living in assisted living. Administrators working in assisted living communities must have a comprehensive understanding of the civil, legal, social, and ethical rights of all assisted living residents. Elders in assisted living communities are vulnerable because of multiple physical and psychosocial problems and thus must be assured that protections needed for basic safety and quality of life.

A STEP-BY-STEP GUIDE TO BECOMING AN ASSISTED LIVING/ RESIDENTIAL CARE ADMINISTRATOR

Aspiring residential care/assisted living administrators must identify a particular path to fulfill their professional goal and obtain a career in LTC administration. While there are different options for students and practitioners, the following guide explores possible steps to becoming a residential care/assisted living administrator.

Step 1: Do you have the passion and drive to serve and work with diverse, older adults who live in residential care/assisted living communities?

Preparing for a career in residential care/assisted living administration can and should start with a desire to serve and work with diverse older adults. Do you have personal experience with older family members and/or friends? Do you have volunteer experience with older neighbors, offering help to older adults in community/senior centers, assisting older adults who live in residential care/assisted living communities or SNF?

Step 2: Do you meet the minimal state regulations for education/training for residential care/assisted living administrators?

Each state sets its own residential care/assisted living regulations and administers its own certification/licensure examination. The NCAL publishes the *Assisted Living State Regulatory Review* on an annual basis; it is a comprehensive report in which you can check the most current regulations for the state where you intend to practice (www.ahcancal.org/Assisted-Living/Policy/Documents/2019_reg_review.pdf). There is no federal requirement for residential care/assisted living administrator certification/licensure at this time.

Specifically, you should check the state regulations for any minimal age requirement (usually 18–21 years of age), minimal education and training requirements (usually a bachelor's degree with field experience) as well as other important qualifications (e.g., Live Scan background check, etc.). Students should focus their search on universities and colleges that offer degrees in gerontology or closely related fields. Many choose to become registered nurses or social workers to gain some clinical training, while others focus more on administrative qualifications in their education and work experience.

Academic programs in gerontology specifically provide the knowledge and experiences students will need to manage daily operations, handle resident requirements, and assist with budgeting. Students should take courses on LTC administration, health administration, and business administration. Administrator-In-Training (AIT) programs or internship placements at a residential care/assisted living community are applied courses that will help students leverage and apply what they learn in the classroom to their work in the field.

Step 3: Do you have a master's degree in gerontology or a related field?

An MA degree in gerontology with a specialization in LTC administration is the preferred path to becoming a residential care/assisted living administrator as it allows students to deepen their knowledge in critical areas and specialize in subjects that are most important to them (e.g., Alzheimer's disease and memory loss enhancement programs).

A master's degree in gerontology or a related field can also set one apart during the interview process. However, students can also enroll in a master's of science degree in gerontology, which can provide them with similar education but with a heavier clinical focus (e.g., infection control and universal precautions).

Step 4: Do you have a professional credential in residential care/assisted living administration?

The penultimate step is becoming certified and/or licensed as a residential care/assisted living administrator. Each state sets its own residential care/assisted living regulations and administers its own certification/licensure examination. The NCAL publishes the *Assisted Living State Regulatory Review* on an annual basis; it is a comprehensive report in which you can check the most current regulations for the state where you intend to practice (www.ahcancal.org/Assisted-Living/Policy/Documents/2019_reg_review.pdf).

In addition to reviewing the state regulations information that is provided by the NCAL report, be very sure to use the link that is listed for the state regulatory website where you intend to practice for additional details on how to prepare and take the state certification/licensure examination in residential care/assisted living administration.

For example, if you go to the *Assisted Living State Regulatory Review* and check for California, you will find the most current regulations summarized by NCAL as well as a link to the California regulatory website (www.ccld.ca.gov). This state regulatory website contains information on "How to Become a Certified Administrator," with specific details on the state-administered exam. Of particular interest to any potential exam applicant is any state news update in relation to the state certification/licensure exam process. At this time, given the current COVID-19 pandemic, the state regulatory web site stated:

"Due to the State of Emergency, the Administrator Exam has been suspended. At this time, the Administrator Certification Section (ACS) is unable to provide the exam electronically. Once you have completed the Initial Certification Training Program (ICTP) and need to take the Administrator Exam, you may apply for a Conditional Administrator Certificate (following existing procedures minus submitting any proof of passing exam) or follow the existing process to request an extension. Extensions will be approved up to 90 days due to the current State of Emergency.

Once the State of Emergency has been lifted, individuals must take and pass the in-person Administrator Examination in order to receive a Non-Conditional (standard) Administrator Certificate. For further information, please see the Community Care Licensing Division homepage Provider Information Notices (https://cdss.ca.gov/portals/9/ccl/acp/2019/becomecertadmin.pdf)." This is valuable information to have as you plan the steps and timeline on how to become credentialed in residential care/assisted living administration.

According to the NAB, it collaborates with some states (e.g., Missouri, Oklahoma, South Carolina) to design and administer their state licensure exams. However, it is very important to note that these state regulatory boards/agencies are the entities (*not* the NAB) that will issue the required LTC licenses once the criteria has been successfully met. In addition, the NAB has indicated that some states (e.g., Alabama) are *not* in the position to offer residential care/assisted living administrator certification/licensure exams (www.nabweb.org/filebin/pdf/NAB_Handbook_October_2019_WEB.pdf).

Since there is *no* federal requirement for residential care/assisted living administrator certification/licensure at this time, it may make sense for individuals in states with *no* residential care/assisted living administrator certification/licensure exams to opt for *elective* national licensure with NAB and/or *elective* national certification with CDAL in order to be able to document their professional credentialing and qualifications in residential care/assisted living administration.

Step 5: How can I pass the certification/licensure exam in residential care/assisted living administration?

Residential care/assisted living administrator certification/licensure indicates that you meet a certain standard of competence and can give you a competitive advantage, more job opportunities, a higher pay scale, and job security. The best advice for passing a residential care/assisted living administrator certification/licensure exam includes, but is not limited to, the following considerations:

1. Are you eligible and qualified to take the exam?

    Determine if you are eligible and qualified to take the state-administered exam, the NAB exam, or the CDAL exam for certification/licensure in residential care/assisted living administration.

2. Are you ready to submit the appropriate application for the exam?

    Prepare for and submit the appropriate application for the state-administered exam, the NAB exam, or CDAL exam for certification/licensure in residential care/assisted living administration with attention to cost and when and where the exam will be administered.

3. Do you understand the exam objectives, questions, and exam format?

    To pass your exam in residential care/assisted living administration, you will need to investigate the exam objectives, questions, and format in order to have a better understanding of what to expect when taking the actual exam. Break the exam objectives into categories to structure studying and cover all the information and state regulations you need to. As for the exam format, is it multiple-choice, multiple-answer, true–false, or a combination of these questions? How many questions are on the exam? What is the length of the exam? What's the passing score? Can you take a brief break and leave the exam room?

4. Do you have time to prepare for the exam?

    Be sure to optimize time management skills in order to make sure you have enough time to study every day. Opt to study in a quiet environment without distractions and use effective study habits to retain all the information better. This will ensure better results and increased chances of passing the exam in residential care/assisted living administration.

5. Do you use multiple resources to study for the exam?

    Collect all the review materials available on residential care/assisted living administration, and be sure that they are current and relevant to the exam. Try not to rely on one source of information; it may diminish your chances of success. In this case, review courses are very helpful because instructors have experience that can provide up-to-date information. A combination of formal education and studying from multiple resources will ensure that you get a balanced review experience and that you are better prepared for your exam.

6. Do you have a strategy to prepare for the exam?

    Do you already have some experience in residential care/assisted living administration, or are you a novice? How much time do you devote to studying in a day? How much study material do you need to go through? To prepare yourself sufficiently, you need the right exam preparation strategy. If you work and need to prepare to take an exam, you should start preparing months in advance. Create daily, weekly, and monthly schedules and stick to them.

7. Does practice make perfect?

    The best preparation for an exam is hands-on training or practical experience because it's the most effective way to get an in-depth understanding of the state regulations in residential care/assisted living administration. Retaining knowledge and recalling it when needed is easy when you understand techniques. Also, you should take practice tests and research older versions of the exam to see which topics and exam questions are always covered. Taking a practice exam will help you detect any weak points that you can address later. Take your time to become familiar with the testing procedure.

8. Will you take the exam the right way?

    When you find yourself in the testing center with the exam in front of you, remember that proper time management is essential. If you spend too much time on some questions, then you won't have enough time to answer the other questions. Divide the total exam time by the number of questions on the exam, and you will get the average time you have to answer each question. Next, do all the easiest questions first and then go back to review the tougher ones. Don't spend too much time on each question. If you cannot answer two or three questions, don't worry because most exams have a certain passing score that's below 100%. Some questions can be tricky, so be sure to read each of them carefully to understand the meaning and identify keywords. This will help you avoid spending too much time on certain questions, which may cause you to run out of time. If you have the time at the end of your exam, go back to double-check your answers.

9. Are you ready for the exam?

    When the test date comes, make sure you are at the testing center at least half an hour early. Have the right identification form with you (i.e., your driver's license and/or passport). Before taking the exam, be sure to de-stress. Performance anxiety comes when you are worried about whether you will be able to perform at your best. Just remind yourself that you are ready to tackle the challenge. If you have covered all exam topics, gone through the practice questions, and studied hard—you should be ready for the exam in residential care/assisted living administration (MyComputerCareer, 2021).

10. A *Review Guide* Makes It Easier

    A *Review Guide* is probably one of the best ways to pass your exam. To pass it successfully, you must put in a lot of work studying the state regulations, *Second Edition*, and *Review Guide*. These resources will provide reliable and in-depth information that will help you study on your own and pass the exam. In this *Review Guide*, you will find over 300 sample test questions from each of the five Domains of Practice. Answers with detailed rationales are provided. The score is based on the number of questions answered correctly; do not leave any of the questions unanswered—guess at the best response if you must. Try taking the sample test questions and see how you do. With practice, you will be primed to pass the exam.

Step 6: How can I maintain recertification/relicensure in residential care/assisted living administration?

Passing your exam is not the last thing you have to do to be a certified/licensed residential care/assisted living administrator. As soon as your certification/licensure arrives, you need to start thinking about maintaining your professional credentials. In order to maintain recertification/relicensure, a residential care/assisted living administrator must obtain Continuing Education Contact Hours based on state regulations. Each state sets its own residential care/assisted living regulations and maintains its own recertification/relicensure requirements (e.g., the number of Continuing Education Contact Hours, how often you need these hours, what topics you need these hours in, etc.). The NCAL publishes the *Assisted Living State Regulatory Review* on an annual basis; it is a comprehensive report in which you can check the most current regulations for your state (www.ahcancal.org/Assisted-Living/Policy/Documents/2019_reg_review.pdf) and how to maintain recertification/relicensure in residential care/assisted living administration.

REFERENCES

Administration on Aging. (2020). *2019 profile of older Americans.* https://acl.gov/sites/default/files/Aging%20and%20Disability%20in%20America/2019ProfileOlderAmericans508.pdf

Allen, J. E. (2004). *Assisted living administration: The knowledge base* (2nd ed.). Springer. https://www.google.com/books/edition/Assisted_Living_Administration/ApsGIsj2jagC?hl=en&gbpv=1&printsec=frontcover

MyComputerCareer. (2021). *What are the best tips for passing a certification exam?* https://www.mycomputercareer.edu/what-are-the-best-tips-for-passing-a-certification-exam/

National Association of Long-Term Care Administrator Boards. (n.d.). *NAB domains of practice.* https://www.nabweb.org/nab-domains-of-practice-2

National Center for Assisted Living. (2019). *2019 assisted living state regulatory review.* Retrieved June 11, 2021, from https://www.ahcancal.org/Assisted-Living/Policy/Documents/2019_reg_review.pdf

Professional Testing, Inc. (2006). *Certification and licensure tests.* https://proftesting.com/test_topics/pdfs/test_types_cert.pdf

Target Health. (2017). *Gerontology, history of medicine.* https://www.targethealth.com/post/gerontology

United Nations, Department of Economic and Social Affairs, Population Division (2019). *World population ageing 2019: Highlights* (ST/ESA/SER.A/430). https://www.un.org/en/development/desa/population/publications/pdf/ageing/WorldPopulationAgeing2019-Highlights.pdf

U.S. Census Bureau. (2011a). *The older population: 2010.* https://www.census.gov/prod/cen2010/briefs/c2010br-09.pdf

U.S. Census Bureau. (2011b). *2010 census shows 65 and older population growing faster than total U.S. population.* https://www.census.gov/newsroom/releases/archives/2010_census/cb11-cn192.html#:~:text=For%20most%20single%20years%20of,compared%20with%20176%2C689%2C%20respectively).

U.S. Census Bureau. (2020). *65 and older population grows rapidly as Baby Boomers age.* https://www.census.gov/newsroom/press-releases/2020/65-older-population-grows.html

Yee-Melichar, D., Flores, C., & Boyle, A. R. (2021). *Assisted living administration and management: Effective practices and model programs in elder care* (2nd ed.). Springer. https://www.springerpub.com/assisted-living-administration-and-management-9780826161949.html

CHAPTER 1

ORGANIZATIONAL MANAGEMENT

1. Long-term care is defined as
   A. personal care
   B. social services
   C. sustained care over 90 days
   D. for persons with chronic conditions or functional limitations
   E. All of the above

2. What is the name of the generation of senior moving into assisted living?
   A. Baby Boomers
   B. Generation X
   C. Generation Z
   D. The Greatest Generation
   E. Millennials

3. Adult Day Care (ADC)
   A. is a way to give caregivers a break
   B. is a place to offer social interaction for seniors
   C. offers meals one to five times per week
   D. can include some medical services
   E. All of the above

4. Which is the fastest growing age group in the country?
   A. 0 to 18
   B. 21 to 30
   C. 31 to 50
   D. 51 to 70
   E. 85 and older

5. How should the quality of care improve in assisted living?
   A. Administrator education
   B. Accountability and oversight
   C. Affordable care
   D. Staffing standards
   E. All of the above

6. Which of the following is <u>not</u> considered a long-term care provider option for seniors?
   A. Senior-themed cruises or hotels
   B. Assisted living
   C. Continuing Care Communities
   D. Adult Day Care
   E. Skilled Nursing

7. The Assisted Living Workgroup in 2003 made the following recommendations for pre admission with the exception of which of the following:
   A. Disclosure of advanced directive
   B. Disclosure of image or identity guidelines
   C. Disclosure of specialized care programs
   D. Disclosure of end-of-life care
   E. Disclosure of the process of assessing residents

8. What percentage of residents in an assisted living facility are older than 85?
   A. 50%
   B. 75%
   C. 60%
   D. 90%
   E. 83%

9. Name the characteristics of residents residing in the assisted living setting. Select all that apply:
   A. Majority of the residents are female
   B. Majority of the residents are non-Hispanic and White
   C. Majority of residents have a chronic condition such as high blood pressure or dementia
   D. 40% of residents require assistance with three or more activities of daily living (ADLs)
   E. All of the above

10. When was the term <u>assisted living</u> first used?
    A. 1969
    B. 35 years ago
    C. 1991
    D. 1965
    E. 2001

11. What will the number of seniors using paid long-term care services be by 2050?
    A. 13 million
    B. 20 million
    C. 27 million
    D. 10 million
    E. Too many to count

12. How many states did not report a regulatory change between 2018 and 2019?
    A. 10
    B. 35
    C. 23
    D. 42
    E. 16

13. Why was the Assisted Living Workgroup formed?
    A. To improve profitability of assisted living homes
    B. To address safety and quality of care issues
    C. To train future administrators
    D. To educate students on assisted living topics
    E. To operate assisted living communities throughout the United States

14. Assisted living has become increasingly popular for the following reasons:
    A. The traditional nursing home option was not an enjoyable environment
    B. Consumers desired an alternative living option that was more home-like
    C. Assisted living options allow for functional capability and autonomy
    D. Assisted living environments allowed for multiple living options from independent living to memory care
    E. All of the above

15. What is the definition of <u>assisted living</u>?
    A. A community that offers room and board with provisions for ADLs
    B. There is no true definition for <u>assisted living</u>
    C. An option for living between one's own home and a nursing home
    D. Housing for the elderly with supportive services
    E. All of the above

16. The Center for Excellence in Assisted Living includes which of the following organizations?
    A. Pioneer Network
    B. Agriforum
    C. Argentum
    D. American Cancer Society
    E. A and D

17. Residents enter assisted living from the following places:
    A. Their home
    B. Skilled Nursing
    C. Hospital
    D. Other assisted living facilities
    E. All of the above

18. Which of these is <u>not</u> considered a Resident Right?
    A. Right to choose your own dentist
    B. Right to practice Buddhism
    C. Right to smoke in home
    D. Right to complain
    E. Right to receive unopened mail

19. Which of the following are considered activities of daily living? Select all that apply.
    A. Bathing and grooming
    B. Medication management
    C. Financial management
    D. Medical and health consulting
    E. A and B

20. What are the typical admission and retention criteria in an assisted living?
    A. Health-related conditions
    B. Functional conditions
    C. Physical function
    D. Cognitive function
    E. All of the above

21. Except for which of the following are provider responsibilities?
    A. Promote an environment of civility
    B. Maintain an environment free of illegal weapons and drugs
    C. Establish and maintain house rules
    D. Involve staff in resident service plans
    E. None of the above; all are provider responsibilities

22. An example of Residents Rights in assisted living would be which of the following?
    A. Right to root for the home team
    B. Right to remain silent
    C. Right to extra ice cream
    D. Right to use image on social media
    E. Right to be treated with respect and dignity

23. What does OSHA do for assisted living?
    A. Allows for employees to use chemicals
    B. Allows for employees to get hurt on the job
    C. Allows for employers to avoid safety inspections
    D. Allows for employees to be free from recognized hazards at work
    E. All of the above

24. Federal nursing home laws require direct care staff to complete how many hours of training prior to direct care?
    A. 40 hours
    B. 16 hours
    C. 75 hours
    D. 80 hours
    E. 8 hours

25. How does the Fair Labor Standards Act benefit assisted living?
    A. Requires pay for overtime
    B. Mandates employee break periods
    C. Established equal pay standards
    D. Mandates employees are paid for training hours
    E. All of the above

26. What are three of the federal statutes that impact assisted living?
    A. Family and Medical Leave Act (FMLA), Social Security Act, Consumer Safety Act
    B. Fair Housing Amendment Act, FMLA, Fair Employment and Housing Act (FEHA)
    C. Federal Emergency Management Agency, Security and Exchange Commission, OSHA
    D. Civil Rights Act of 1991, Rehabilitation Act of 1973, FMLA
    E. NCAA, MLBA, NFL

27. What percentage of seniors will need long-term care for <5 years?
    A. 86%
    B. 78%
    C. 14%
    D. 33%
    E. 63%

28. Zimmerman and Sloan (2007) describe various models relative to size and unit types. Which is not considered the three-part typology?
    A. New model, large facility
    B. Board and Care
    C. 16 beds or more older than 1987
    D. 16 beds or less
    E. None of the above

29. The Americans with Disabilities Act affects assisted living in which two ways?
    A. Building and staff
    B. Residents and staff
    C. Building and residents
    D. Residents and visitors
    E. Visitors and staff

30. For-profit investors are interested in the assisted living industry. Which of the following are not areas of concerns?
    A. High returns on investments
    B. Quality service providers
    C. Long-term stability
    D. Legal risks
    E. Fewer number of seniors needing care

31. State philosophy on regulation typically allows for privacy, autonomy, and community decision-making. What kind of philosophy does this represent?
    A. A regulation-centered philosophy to keep residents safe
    B. A rule-centric philosophy to increase lawsuits and legal consequences
    C. A philosophy which is consumer focused and resident-centric
    D. A bureaucratic philosophy with strong oversight and enforcement
    E. A laissez-fair approach

32. What is an example of the future landscape of assisted living?
    A. Granny flats
    B. Green House Project
    C. Residential care facilities
    D. Stonewall Gardens
    E. Unknown

33. What are the two state regulatory systems Erin Carlson described in 2005?
    A. Single level or multi level
    B. Laissez-faire or universal
    C. Holistic or binary
    D. Democratic or republican
    E. Corporation or private interests

34. Which of the following is <u>not</u> considered an "affiliation" assisted living community?
    A. Religious interest
    B. LGBTQ supportive
    C. Ethnic group
    D. Political affiliation

35. Which of the following is <u>not</u> one of the descriptive benefits of "Memory Care"?
    A. Environment that promotes independence within a secured setting
    B. Environment that provides specialized training, activities and philosophies to aid residents with memory impairment
    C. Environment that encourages limited staff and resident interaction
    D. Environment to enhance the life of someone with dementia
    E. Environment to provide a safe space for someone with a memory impairment

36. What is a "board-and-care" model?
    A. Large community with multiple amenities
    B. High-privacy accommodations
    C. Small group home
    D. Home located in large urban area
    E. Hotel-like

37. How do not-for-profit assisted living communities make money?
    A. Resident rent
    B. Donations
    C. Fundraising events
    D. Reduce staffing levels
    E. A, B, and C

38. What is <u>not</u> an intervention for a specialized memory care community?
    A. Holistic environment
    B. Safety restraints to limit resident injury
    C. Person-centered care
    D. Medications to treat aggressive behaviors
    E. B and D

39. What is the standardized model of care in assisted living?
    A. Personalized care
    B. Levels of care
    C. No official standardized model
    D. All services included
    E. Only when needed

40. Why have there been historical problems with resident agreements?
    A. Did not include discharge criteria
    B. Did not explain how or why costs for care assistance changes
    C. Did not describe services not provided by facility
    D. Did not address grievance procedures
    E. All of the above

41. The service models in assisted living can include which of the following:
    A. Hospitality
    B. Board and care
    C. Dementia care only
    D. Large scale
    E. All of the above

42. How many states do not have an option for using Medicaid to fund services in assisted living?
    A. 8
    B. 15
    C. 25
    D. 2
    E. 35

43. What does <u>aging in place</u> mean?
    A. The person changes, but the environment stays the same
    B. A person does not have to move if care needs change
    C. Needs can be accommodated in the living environment
    D. Boomers like to stay in the same place
    E. All of the above

44. Which is <u>not</u> a component of a board and care model?
    A. A large number of staff
    B. Small home size
    C. Residential neighborhood
    D. Limited independence and privacy
    E. May have home health or hospice services from third-party vendors

45. What similar objective does an administrator have in a for-profit or not-for-profit assisted living community?
    A. Drive margin to make more revenue
    B. Reduce costs by minimizing staff levels
    C. Complete daily reports and holding staff meetings
    D. Organizing a plan that will be better than other organizations
    E. Avoid regulatory problems by limited communication to state agencies

46. What is not one of the limitations of aging in place in assisted living?
    A. Hospice or end-of-life needs
    B. State regulations
    C. Care model
    D. Community discretion
    E. Medical model

47. A "hospitality model" in assisted living does <u>not</u> include which of the following?
    A. Residential setting
    B. Hotel services
    C. Meals provided
    D. Medications provided
    E. High level of privacy

48. Which of the following is <u>not</u> a benefit of aging in place?
    A. Resident dignity
    B. Socialization
    C. Supportive services
    D. Residents never have to leave the apartment
    E. Hospice services available to support end-of-life care

49. Why does a "hospitality model" experience a high turnover rate?
    A. Lower level of care
    B. No RN on staff
    C. Laundry not folded properly
    D. All of the above
    E. A and B

50. Why would a resident desire to live in an "affiliated" assisted living community?
    A. Common language
    B. Religious preference
    C. Cultural acceptance
    D. Common values
    E. All of the above

51. What is <u>not</u> one of the conclusions made about larger model communities?
    A. Services are not able to meet the needs of residents through end of life
    B. They are valued by customers
    C. They offer a wide variety of services
    D. They are largely unaffordable to moderate- or low-income seniors
    E. They allow for resident independence and privacy

CHAPTER 2

HUMAN RESOURCES MANAGEMENT

1. In the example provided, Meadowlark Hills Retirement Community in Manhattan, Kansas, holds Learning Circles _____ to address concerns and work through problems?
   A. annually
   B. monthly
   C. weekly
   D. daily

2. In which state would you be able to be an administrator at the age of 18?
   A. Rhode Island
   B. Ohio
   C. Utah
   D. Washington
   E. California

3. An effective interview will successfully match the best available candidate to the specific position. Identify some characteristics of an effective interview. Select all that apply.
   A. Carefully planned questions prepared in advance
   B. Offer applicant something to drink
   C. Tour of the facility
   D. Realistic perspective of the job, both favorable and unfavorable information
   E. A, C, and D
   F. All of the above

4. What component of the recruitment process involves the elimination of unqualified applicants from the recruitment pool?
   A. Selection
   B. Screening
   C. Hiring
   D. Planning
   E. Projection

5. In the state of New York, administrators must meet which of the following requirements:
   A. 21 years of age
   B. Three letters of recommendations proving good moral character
   C. Varying levels of education and experience
   D. All of the above
   E. None of the above

6. Direct care worker jobs are viewed by the public as unpleasant and poor paying, which makes staff recruitment challenging. In order to recruit direct care workers and improve the image of the senior care industry, what must we address?
   A. Media reports
   B. Family dynamics
   C. Ageism
   D. A and C
   E. All of the above

7. Which staff, as the "eyes and ears" of the care system, should be included in direct care planning?
   A. Night staff
   B. Administrators
   C. Direct care staff
   D. Outside contractors
   E. Medical Technicians

8. What are the steps in the recruitment process?
   A. Planning, searching, screening, hiring
   B. Planning, searching, screening, selection and hiring, maintaining applicant pool
   C. Searching, screening, selection, hiring
   D. Planning, screening, searching, selection and hiring, maintaining applicant pool
   E. Planning, searching, screening, selection and hiring, maintaining applicant pool

9. What are some methods recruiting candidates from external sources?
   A. Community job fairs
   B. Advertisements in professional newsletters
   C. Community Outreach Programs
   D. Referrals from employees and friends
   E. All of the above

10. Individuals with high levels of disability and complex health conditions receive long-term care in home and community-based settings, increasing the skill demands both for family caregivers and paid workers. What must direct care workers receive in order to reduce high rates of staff injury and high rates of turnovers?
    A. Adequate days off
    B. Staff training
    C. Health benefits
    D. Adequate pay
    E. Paid time off

11. Which component of the recruitment process identifies the importance of advance knowledge of trends in the industry? (The Department of Labor and the Employment Security Commission may also be a source of information to consider in the planning phase.)
    A. Planning
    B. Hiring
    C. Screening
    D. Projections
    E. None of the above

12. In an interview, which of the following is legal to ask an applicant?
    A. A person's religion
    B. Applicant's education history
    C. A person's age
    D. Childcare arrangements
    E. Childbearing plans

13. Who is responsible for projecting the resident needs of the community and identifying the personnel requirements necessary to meet those needs?
    A. Facility administrator
    B. Charge nurse
    C. Staff supervisor
    D. Caregiver
    E. Family members

14. Administrators in this state must complete only 12 hours of continuing education every 2 years on topics related to assisted living:
    A. Alabama
    B. New York
    C. Florida
    D. Iowa
    E. South Carolina

15. Which of the following trends make hiring and recruiting staff a challenge in assisted living communities.
    A. Low wage and benefits
    B. Ageism
    C. Hard working conditions
    D. A lack of training
    E. All of the above

16. What is the minimum age requirement for an administrator in California?
    A. 21
    B. 25
    C. 22
    D. 30
    E. 18

17. What is the benefit recruiting staff from within an organization?
    A. Improved staff morale and loyalty
    B. Increased efficiency
    C. A and B
    D. None of the above
    E. All of the above

18. Assisted living administrators must understand the responsibilities involved with the job, the tasks involved with the job, and the background (i.e., education and experience) necessary to complete the job. What component of the recruitment process is this?
    A. Planning
    B. Projections
    C. Job description
    D. Screening

19. According to the Justice in Aging study, which of the following is not considered one of the characteristics that should be considered when developing dementia training requirements?
    A. Highly detailed training objectives
    B. Outcome-based curriculum with examinations requiring a demonstration that competencies have been mastered
    C. Requirements for continuing education in addition to pre service training
    D. Only state licensing officials should develop training content and design of competency evaluations to avoid bias

20. Which of the following describes Justice in Aging?
    A. A National Advocacy group started in 1972
    B. A National Advocacy Group that identified 18 general approaches to memory care in 1972
    C. In 2015, identified Washington State as one state with strong models of dementia training
    D. A and C

21. Which of the following has not been described goals of the Learning Circles?
    A. Encourages quiet people to talk
    B. Encourages talkative people to listen
    C. Majority rule in decision-making when no consensus develops
    D. Fosters a sense of trust and connection between participants

22. In its report, *Assuring Quality in Assisted Living: Guidelines for Federal and State Policy, State Regulations, and Operations*, the Assisted Living Work Group (2003) included which of the following?
    A. All staff shall have specific orientation relevant to their specific job assignments and responsibilities
    B. There should be appropriate interaction with residents and family members
    C. Contract staff should receive an orientation on topics relevant to their job, including orientation of the facility's fire, life safety, and emergency disaster plans
    D. All of the above

23. As outlined in the textbook, which of the following have not been observed or reported by government agencies and advocates as being a concern for a lack of proper training in assisted living communities?
    A. Insufficient and undertrained staff, low pay rates and high staff turnover
    B. Despite laws and regulations requiring certain minimum staff training, specifics of the training are often left to the individual communities
    C. Lack of number of certified nursing assistants working in assisted living
    D. Inadequate resources to enforcement and oversight of assisted living and inadequate staffing and staff training requirements

24. Which of the following describes the Long-Term Community Coalition?
    A. It is a for-profit organization with altruistic aims
    B. While dedicated to improving quality of care, and quality of life for seniors and those with disabilities, the coalition members could not find common agreement for training best practices
    C. It was dedicated to improving quality of care, quality of life, and dignity for elderly and people with disabilities in nursing homes, assisted living communities, and other residential settings
    D. In 2012 it struggled to find common ground on barely three training best practices

25. Which of the following is/are <u>not</u> generally accepted examples of direct staff training subjects? Select all that apply.
    A. Principles of assisted living
    B. Personal/direct care skills
    C. Hygiene
    D. Mental health/emotional/behavioral needs
    E. Understanding financial reimbursement sources for assisted living
    F. Restraints

26. What are job descriptions utilized to establish?
    A. Salary ranges
    B. Performance expectations
    C. Recruitment plan
    D. A, B, and C
    E. None of the above

27. How might an administrator recognize the value of each employee?
    A. Call each employee by name
    B. Involve staff in the interview process
    C. Listen to the concerns of staff
    D. Provide opportunity for cross over in different departments
    E. All of the above

28. What strategy is utilized when the administrator encourages employees to participate in the development of standards for in-services, attendance, scheduling, routines, and policies and allowing for peer input at job performance reviews?
    A. Peer review
    B. Career ladders
    C. Employee assistance program
    D. None of the above
    E. All of the above

29. What program could the administrator implement to acknowledge employees for their performance? The administrator should make sure that every department on every shift, part-time and full-time, are included.
    A. Display special postings
    B. Employee of the Month
    C. Employee of the Year
    D. B and C
    E. All of the above

30. Paraprofessional Healthcare Institute (PHI) promotes quality direct care jobs as the foundation for quality care. Identify strategies for success growing a strong direct care workforce. Select all that apply.
    A. Promote peer support
    B. Recognize and reward staff
    C. Ensure effective supervision
    D. A and B
    E. All of the above

31. How might an administrator create a positive work experience?
    A. Gain respect
    B. Ensure adequate supplies for the entire community
    C. Establish a comprehensive system of corrective actions that are enforced consistently across disciplines and shifts
    D. Develop excellent and efficient training programs
    E. A and D
    F. All of the above

32. Administrators should pay close attention to employees at risk for leaving employment at the present time. What are some warning signs of potential turnover?
    A. Low pay
    B. Unexplained absences
    C. Visibly unhappy
    D. Rejection for promotion
    E. B, C, and D
    F. All of the above

33. To understand the community's retention challenges, what should the administrators review with managers and department heads on a regular basis?
    A. Negative turnover
    B. Positive turnover
    C. A and B
    D. Staff training and education
    E. None of the above

34. What extrinsic factors are associated with staff retention?
    A. Low rates of professional staff turnover
    B. Employee recognition
    C. Clean, safe work environments
    D. Higher staff ratio
    E. All of the above

35. What can larger statewide or national organizations have to offer that differs from smaller associations?
    A. Strategically planned advocacy program
    B. Professional contacts
    C. Senior care referrals
    D. Community education
    E. C and D

36. The Hospital and Healthcare Compensation Service reported turnover across all assisted living positions declined from 34.96% to what percentage in 2019?
    A. 31.71%
    B. 31.75%
    C. 32.4%
    D. 31.79%
    E. 32.8%

37. Unexplained absences, reduced interest in the job, life events such as childbirth, death, or divorce are warning signs for potential _____.
    A. positive turnover
    B. staff turnover
    C. staff retention
    D. A and B
    E. None of the above

38. What is the least expensive approach to expressing staff appreciation?
    A. Acknowledging staff with a plaque
    B. Providing staff with lunch
    C. Publishing the staff performance in a company newsletter
    D. Saying "thank you"
    E. Monetary bonus at the end of the year

39. Extrinsic factors associated with staff turnover will aid the administrator in developing strategies to improve retention over time. What are some extrinsic factors associated with staff turnover?
    A. Wage and benefits
    B. Excessive workload
    C. Inadequate job training
    D. A lack of respect
    E. All of the above

40. How does a reward system benefit staff?
    A. Creates positive working condition
    B. Increases wage and benefits
    C. Promotes staff retention
    D. A and C
    E. None of the above

41. Direct care staff are the "eyes and ears" of assisted living. Administrators should consider input from caregivers. Which is the best approach? Select all that apply.
    A. Request and accept input from employees for changes to policies and procedures
    B. Ask staff to share their problems and successes
    C. Seek the participation of direct care staff in resident specific concerns, such as behavioral or feeding problems
    D. Ask staff to request information from family regarding the resident
    E. A, B, and C
    F. All of the above

42. What program should assisted living communities have in place to create morale?
    A. Special recognition/appreciation
    B. Health benefits
    C. Staff training
    D. Provide food at staff meetings

43. To understand the community's retention challenges, the administrator should review turn-over daily with managers. What should administrators aim for?
    A. Promote positive turnover
    B. Encourage staff support
    C. Maintain positive turnover
    D. A and C
    E. All of the above

44. According to research, what is employee empowerment associated with in assisted living?
    A. Morale
    B. Employee productivity
    C. Job satisfaction
    D. B and C
    E. A and C
    F. All of the above

45. What are some incentives an administrator can offer to promote staff retention?
    A. Provide inexpensive vending items
    B. Sponsor employee sports teams or purchase shirts printed with the community logo
    C. Pay an allowance for uniforms, negotiate discounts for employees at local uniforms shops
    D. Arrange for discounted purchases of bus passes
    E. Provide free coffee or tea in the employee lounge
    F. All of the above

46. In California, which topics are required annually for direct care staff caring for residents with dementia? Select all that apply.
    A. Positive therapeutic interventions and activities such as exercise, sensory stimulation, activities of daily living, and social, recreational, and rehabilitative activities
    B. Common problems such as wandering, aggression, and inappropriate sexual behavior
    C. End-of-life issues, including hospice
    D. Dietary needs
    E. A, B, and C
    F. All of the above

47. According to California's Residential Care Facilities for the Elderly (RCFE) Reform Act, what minimum required knowledge must administrators in California possess?
    A. Ability to maintain or supervise the maintenance of financial and other records
    B. Knowledge of the requirements for providing care and supervision appropriate to the residents
    C. A only
    D. A and B
    E. None of the above

48. What are some of the benefits in joining a professional association? Select all that apply.
    A. Education
    B. Alliances
    C. Community service
    D. Networking
    E. All of the above

49. In California, how many additional hours must direct care staff providing care to residents with dementia receive?
    A. 4 hours
    B. 6 hours
    C. 10 hours
    D. 8 hours
    E. 2 hours

50. When offering continuing education and professional development opportunities to employees, which group or groups must administrators acknowledge in the workforce?
    A. Baby Boomers
    B. Millennials
    C. Gen X
    D. Gen Y
    E. A, B, and C

51. What age are the Gen Xers?
    A. 20s and 30s
    B. 40s and 50s
    C. 30s and 40s
    D. 50s and 60s

52. How would an administrator support continuing education to their employees?
    A. Provide more funding for access to continuing education
    B. Provide required staff coverage
    C. A
    D. A and B
    E. None of the above

53. When considering Millennials in the workforce, what should assisted living administrators understand about this group?
    A. They are advancing in their careers and beginning to take on leadership roles at their companies
    B. They value engagement at work, which consists highly of training and personal development in their jobs
    C. They are new to senior care and therefore continuing education will be important in their career advancement
    D. A and B
    E. A, B, and C

54. In California, what legislative bill expanded and specified continuing education requirements for staff in assisted living communities?
    A. SB 914
    B. SB 911
    C. AB 911
    D. AB 914
    E. SB 912

55. Who plays a key role in ensuring that continuing education has a positive effect throughout the community?
    A. Caregivers
    B. Team lead
    C. Administrators
    D. Continuing education provider
    E. None of the above

56. What is the focus on improving and redesigning healthcare systems?
    A. System improvements
    B. Emphasis on teamwork
    C. Collaboration across members of health professions
    D. B and C
    E. A and C
    F. All of the above

57. What is one factor hindering the effectiveness of continuing education in long-term care?
    A. Resistance to change
    B. Changing resident population with harder care needs
    C. Not enough on-the-job training
    D. A, B, and C
    E. A and B

58. In California, direct care staff must receive education on which topics related to senior care and aging?. Select all that apply.
    A. Cultural competency and sensitivity in issues relating to the underserved aging LGBT community
    B. Building and fire safety and appropriate response to emergencies
    C. Residents' rights and personal rights
    D. Recognizing the signs and symptoms of dementia in individuals
    E. All of the above

59. Why is attending conferences an important aspect of continuing education for both administrators and direct care staff?
    A. It provides continuing education credits towards different certificates and licenses
    B. It provides an opportunity for advocating for senior care
    C. It provides a networking opportunity for strong professional connections
    D. A and C
    E. A and B

60. Baby Boomers (a generation 76 million strong) are reaching the traditional retirement age, but many are continuing to work well into what age range?
    A. 60s and 70s
    B. 80s
    C. 50s
    D. 90s

61. In California, what did the RCFE Reform Act of 2014 aim to accomplish?
    A. Focus on improving care
    B. Empower residents
    C. Provide the licensing agency with new tools to ensure compliance with regulatory standards
    D. A and B
    E. All of the above

62. What are the benefits of continuing education utilizing a classroom-style format?
    A. Getting real-time questions answered by the facilitator or by a peer
    B. The ability to troubleshoot among professionals
    C. Expanding your network of other providers
    D. A and C
    E. All of the above

63. Which statement is considered to be true?
    A. Healthcare in the United States is the costliest systems in the world but with poorer outcomes than many other developed and developing countries
    B. Healthcare in the United States is the costliest systems in the world but produces better outcomes than many other developed and developing countries
    C. Healthcare in the United States is the costliest systems in the world because it utilizes the latest technology in healthcare than many other developed and developing countries
    D. The United States offers the most advanced procedures and treatments in healthcare and therefore produces better outcomes than many other developed and developing countries

64. Which professional is responsible for oversight of medical care for residents, including diagnosis and management of illnesses, prescription management for all chronic and acute illnesses, and prescriptions for medical treatments as needed?
    A. Physician
    B. Pharmacist
    C. Registered nurse
    D. Physician assistant
    E. Social worker

65. Who would be part of the interprofessional team? Select all that apply.
    A. Dietician
    B. Pharmacist
    C. Social worker
    D. Physician
    E. Dentist
    F. All of the above

66. In which areas has <u>moderate need for knowledge</u> been identified by most administrators. Select all that apply.
    A. Biology of aging
    B. Hospice regulations
    C. Death and dying
    D. Dementia regulations
    E. All of the above

67. What prompted government-based incentives for healthcare providers to improve quality and safety outcomes, placing the patient at the center of value-based care rather than volume-based care?
    A. Patient Protection and Affordable Care Act
    B. Patient Care Act
    C. Patient Care and Affordable Care Act
    D. Patient Protection and Collaborative Care Act
    E. None of the above

68. What external forces are facilitating the change in the U.S. healthcare delivery?
    A. Increase in quality improvement measures and additional patient safety initiatives
    B. An increased need for improved care transitions and healthcare practice redesign
    C. Escalating healthcare costs
    D. Initiation of federal and state healthcare policies
    E. C and E
    F. All of the above

69. What is the registered nurse in the interprofessional team responsible for? Select all that apply.
    A. Delegates decisions and treatment recommendations to licensed practical nurses and nursing assistants
    B. Responsible for safe delegation of care to licensed vocational nurses as well as unlicensed personnel such as nursing assistants
    C. Oversight and evaluation of direct patient care delivery including patient assessments, hygiene, mobility, and personal care
    D. Oversight of medication administration
    E. Provides direct supervision to licensed vocational nurses and nursing assistants
    F. All of the above

70. Chaplains are part of the interprofessional team. What are some services a chaplain may provide? Select all that apply.
    A. Assessment of individualized care plans for elders
    B. Facilitation of religious rituals and prayers
    C. Provision of leadership within the healthcare setting
    D. Provision of education and consultation for patients and staff
    E. B and D
    F. All of the above

71. Which professional in the interprofessional team is viewed as a leader in rehabilitation allowing patients with disease or chronic health conditions, impaired body functions, injuries, or activity limitations to improve their functional status?
    A. Occupational therapist
    B. Speech therapist
    C. Physical therapist
    D. Physician
    E. Nurse

72. What is the critical element that must exist among healthcare professionals in an interprofessional approach?
    A. Communication
    B. Mutual understanding
    C. Mutual respect
    D. Leadership
    E. All of the above

73. What factors are responsible for the adverse health system and patient outcomes?
    A. A lack of teamwork
    B. Inadequate communication
    C. Limited collaboration
    D. A and C
    E. All of the above

74. What is identified as a major source of medical errors and was connected to quality and safety problems?
    A. A lack of teamwork
    B. Poor communication
    C. Limited collaboration
    D. A and B
    E. All of the above

75. What did the 2016 reauthorization of the Older Americans Act of 1965 include in approved health screenings?
    A. Oral health
    B. Dementia care
    C. Mental health
    D. Physical health
    E. All of the above

76. Research evidence has proven that the use of collaborative practice is shown to decrease which of the following? Select all that apply.
    A. Patient illness outcomes
    B. Staff turnover
    C. Clinical error rates
    D. Mortality rates
    E. Hospital readmission rates
    F. All of the above

CHAPTER 3

BUSINESS AND FINANCIAL MANAGEMENT

1. Regarding medications in assisted living, which of the following is <u>not</u> fair to say?
   A. Most states rely on an assumption that residents retain the mental capacity to give consent to the administration of medications, and the physical ability to take medications on their own
   B. Because most states assume the resident retains some capacity to know what medications they are taking, facilities don't face as much liability concerns whenever a medication mistake is made, because the assisted living community is merely "helping" the resident.
   C. If facilities employ nurses, they should carefully supervise the nursing performance, as the appropriate care standard may be higher than a customary assisted living standard
   D. As a result state laws trying to be very precise in limitations on what exactly can and cannot be done with medications, medication administration has become a fairly confusing process where the law is sometimes inadequately matched to reality

2. Which is not one of the four distinct process steps for total quality management (TQM)?
   A. A belief in the process working
   B. Continuous improvement
   C. The process should have an aesthetic property
   D. Limited scope of each leader in the process
   E. Understanding how the product is used

3. How many items should an effective business plan include (at a minimum):
   A. 3
   B. 8
   C. 7
   D. 5
   E. 15

4. Which item is <u>not</u> one of the components of a strategic business plan?
   A. The time frame of the business plan
   B. The monetary resources required
   C. The level of experience and education of the CEO
   D. The key business strategies
   E. How the business will be operated

5. What term is used repeatedly in the literature of Churchman (1968) and von Bertalanfy (1968) to describe the concept and creation of an organization?
   A. Program
   B. System
   C. Conceptualize
   D. Pragmatize
   E. Locate

6. In an operational plan, managers must maintain control, effectiveness, and focus within the organization. Which is not one of the control points of the operational plan?
   A. Resource utilization
   B. Service program
   C. Process management
   D. Quality controls
   E. Marketing program

7. A change process occurs after the implementation of an evaluation plan. Which element is not one the essential components of the change process?
   A. Must include a basis for improvement
   B. Must focus on a service process or their outcomes
   C. Must provide ways to adapt to changing conditions
   D. Must have an adaptive process for the organization
   E. Must ensure that past failures remain constant

8. Which is not one of the constraints to management and operations?
   A. Budget
   B. Size of the organization
   C. An ideal management approach
   D. Management should fit the needs of the organization
   E. Goals of the organization

9. Why is it important to determine the effectiveness of the marketing plan?
   A. To meet the goals of the community
   B. To determine if the methods used are cost effective
   C. To determine how are we doing compared to our competitors
   D. To ensure we are continually improving our marketing efforts
   E. All of the above

10. Of the following, which is the only true statement about "causation" in a legal case?
    A. As discussed in the text, there are three types of causation: factual causation, natural event incidents, and legal causation
    B. Injuries of the victim must have been caused, at least in part, by the breach of the duty of care that occurred
    C. Assisted living providers should therefore avoid documenting all instances where a resident's risk of injury was assessed and communicated to the resident or their legal decision maker as it may be used against them
    D. Legal causation, also known as proximate causation, should not be confused with the chain of events between the perpetrator's actions or nonactions and the damages at issue but rather what a statute or regulation specifically calls for

11. Which management theory was developed by the Department of Defense in the early 1960s?
    A. Deming Method
    B. Six Sigma
    C. PPBS
    D. BRP
    E. MBO

12. A participatory management style includes which of the following:
    A. Self-management
    B. Limited responsibility
    C. Low value on knowledge of product
    D. Consensus
    E. A and D

13. Which of the following fairly describes the benefits of cash-basis accounting?
    A. It does not demand as many bookkeeping records
    B. Items such as accrued income, accrued expenses, depreciation, expense accounting, revenues, and deductions are <u>not</u> included
    C. It allows companies to be more profitable because they have less accounting overhead
    D. A and B

14. Which management theory stemmed from Maslow's "hierarchy of needs"?
    A. Bureaucratic method
    B. Deming method
    C. Scientific method
    D. Theory Z
    E. TQM

15. How does Buttaro (1994) define <u>management</u>?
    A. Both science and art
    B. Both savvy and sophistication
    C. Both hard work and luck
    D. Both effort and intelligence
    E. None of the above

16. Which of the management theories reflected "reductionism" as a principle?
    A. Bureaucratic method
    B. Deming method
    C. Scientific method
    D. Theory Z
    E. TQM

17. Which management theory takes a top-down chain of command principle?
    A. Theory Z
    B. Theory X
    C. Deming method
    D. Bureaucratic method
    E. Zero defects

18. All of the following statements describe "accrual accounting," except for:
    A. It is the primary accounting method used by assisted living communities (especially large assisted living communities and those communities that are part of a nationwide chain)
    B. Information that is provided can be developed into more meaningful data, giving senior management a more detailed and expanded picture of the overall obligations and prospects
    C. One drawback is that because it is so much more complicated than cash-basis accounting, it decreases the chances of an exact measurement of net income and loss
    D. Recognition of all revenues in the time period they are earned and of all expenses when they are actually incurred

19. As outlined in the textbook, which of the following does not describe Tort Law?
    A. Area of law governing people's relationships with the government regulators, law enforcement, and the courts
    B. A "tort" is committed any time a person or a business violates a basic expectation of a civil relationship, generally speaking, between one another
    C. Examples of torts include battery, slander, medical malpractice, and "personal injury" lawsuits
    D. The key elements to tort law are (a) a civil wrong against a person or property and (b) prosecuted by the victim or their representative

20. Please select the one statement that is not fair to say about a profit and loss statement (or income statement)?
    A. To portray the results of the financial operations in the terms of the amount of revenues the communities has earned
    B. Includes current assets (assets consumed in less than 1 year) such as cash, short-term investments (interest and dividends), patient accounts receivables, inventory
    C. The statement of expenses should not be reported in compartmentalized fashion but in lump sums so managers and officers can see how the entire operations is doing
    D. Includes the amount of expenses the communities has incurred which includes current liabilities (obligations to be paid in 1 year or less), such as accounts payable for vendors, wages/salaries, and taxes

21. "Plan–Do–Study–Act" is the basis for which management theory?
    A. Bureaucratic method
    B. Deming method
    C. Management by organization method
    D. Theory Z
    E. TQM

22. Administration is a separate function from management. What is not one of the service generally provided by administration?
    A. Personnel support and services
    B. Control of flow of money
    C. Informational technology
    D. Interfacing with governmental units
    E. Payroll, billing, and controlling receivables

23. Which of the following is fair to say about resident falls in assisted living?
    A. Preventing falls is made difficult due to a tension between resident safety, on one hand, and allowing resident autonomy, on the other
    B. If appropriate care measures were put in place, assisted living communities would be sure to not have any unwanted falls
    C. Facilities should carefully document its resident fall care plans and be sure to note residents' acceptance or refusal of recommended fall prevention techniques
    D. A and C

24. Which of the following is not fair to say about resident falls in assisted living?
    A. Falls are considered a "standard of care" issue
    B. State laws usually prohibit restraining residents in assisted living but do not set any specific care standards for preventing falls
    C. The law does not require that falls be prevented; it rather expects "reasonable measures" will be undertaken to minimize them at all times
    D. Falls are a "strict liability" issue, so if someone falls, you should expect an automatic citation

25. Which of the following is not an element of a contract?
    A. Offer and acceptance
    B. Consideration
    C. Trust
    D. Capacity

26. All of the following statements describe "remedies" for tort actions, except for:
    A. They generally fall within one of two categories: monetary and equitable relief
    B. Monetary remedies are first focused on punishing the operator and only secondarily making a victim whole
    C. The victim is entitled to all reasonably foreseeable financial damages, including lost wages, medical expenses, and the replacement value of damaged property
    D. There are two main forms of equitable relief: injunctions and specific performance

27. Generally speaking, all of the following are possible grounds for eviction except for which one?
    A. The facility is closing
    B. The resident's medical needs exceed what can be provided by the facility
    C. The resident violates the terms of the admission agreement or other documented rules of the facility
    D. Resident and/or family members complain a lot

28. As outlined in the textbook, which of the following does not describe accounting systems?
    A. Accounting is the system that accumulates data of quantitative nature relating to the activities taking place in the communities
    B. The accounting system should be able to collect data such as the number of admissions, readmissions, resident transfers (upgrades/downgrades), and discharges in order to help senior management perform their strategic planning
    C. To be transparent and to honor resident's rights, the "communication" aspect of accounting corresponds with the reporting of detailed accounting information and presenting to the residents and their families at least once a year so they can rest assured the community is sustainable
    D. Interpretation responds to the analysis of the information (key financial ratios and trends) in order to assist senior management in making correct financial decisions of the assisted living community

29. Which of the following is <u>not</u> fair to say about balance sheets?
    A. By definition, a balance sheet will never show an assisted living community's to have its total liabilities greater than its total assets; otherwise, it couldn't be called a balance sheet
    B. It is usually prepared and reported monthly, quarterly, and annually
    C. It is used to depict the entire financial operation of the communities in terms of its assets, liabilities, and capital (stockholder's equity) at a given period
    D. The sum of invested capital from owners and retained profit is called <u>owners' equity</u>

30. What is <u>not</u> one of Likert's four types of leadership?
    A. Collegial
    B. Exploitive authoritative
    C. Benevolent authoritative
    D. Consultative
    E. Participative

31. Select the one statement that best describes a resident accounts receivable report:
    A. It provides the fiscal operations from the inventory control perspective, knowing what supplies are to be received for resident benefit. It includes only third-party suppliers (food vendors, medical supply vendors). Furthermore, it indicates the effectiveness of the community's process for receiving supplies
    B. It provides the fiscal operations from the income perspective. It includes only income from residents (cash) and third-party payers (state Medicaid, commercial long-term insurance). Furthermore, it indicates the effectiveness of the community's collection and billing procedures
    C. It provides the nonfiscal operations from the income perspective. It includes only income from residents (cash) but not third-party payers (state Medicaid, commercial long-term insurance) since they are not private funds.

CHAPTER 4

ENVIRONMENTAL MANAGEMENT

1. In addition to state regulations governing the life safety of residents, which do they also govern?
   A. Number of staff per shift
   B. Safety trainings for staff
   C. Safety trainings for residents
   D. A and B
   E. B and C

2. The updated Life Safety Codes addressed two main concepts: (1) Larger buildings are more difficult to evacuate and require _____, and (2) occupants who are difficult to move and evacuate will require _____
   A. more fire protection; more built in fire protection
   B. more fire protection; more assistive devices
   C. automatic sprinkler systems; more built in fire protection
   D. Both A and C

3. After a disaster, it is important to help residents through the recovery process by
   A. recovering personal possessions and making residents feel more at home
   B. talking about the disaster and sharing feelings, focusing on personal needs such as sleep, nutrition and medication, and returning to daily routines
   C. not discussing the disaster as it may trigger feelings of fear and anxiety
   D. returning to daily operations to create normalcy

4. In the event of a power outage, what should administrators do?
   A. Arrange transportation to have all residents to be transported off-site
   B. For those who are ambulatory, ask residents to self-evacuate to a family or friends house
   C. Have an emergency generator and emergency equipment readily available
   D. All of the above

5. Hallways in assisted living facilities must be able to accommodate equipment such as _____ and have a minimum of _____ of clearance must be maintained in hallways.
   A. oxygen tanks; 36 inches
   B. wheelchairs; 50 inches
   C. oxygen tanks; 60 inches
   D. hospital beds; 60 inches

6. What is essential in successfully implementing an emergency plan?
   A. Effective communication and accessibility of the plan
   B. Step-by-step written instructions in the plan
   C. Following all Life Safety Codes
   D. None of the above

7. When evacuating it's a good idea to
   A. tell everyone to remain calm and evacuate one person at a time to reduce anxiety and chaos
   B. evacuate close friends or roommates together to reduce stress and anxiety
   C. evacuate the entire building at once to bring everyone to safety
   D. have staff lead the way for residents and evacuate first

8. _____ are created by experts in fire safety and regularly updated to reflect current standards of fire safety professionals
   A. Building regulations
   B. Life Safety Codes
   C. Safety regulations
   D. Fire protection codes

9. If you must evacuate during an emergency, who should be evacuated first?
   A. Residents who are able to ambulate on their own
   B. Residents requiring the most help
   C. Residents in wheelchairs
   D. Everyone should evacuate at the same time

10. International codes for building safety and fire protection have been adopted by how many U.S. states?
    A. 50
    B. 25
    C. 16
    D. 44

11. In assisted living facilities, those with disabilities must have paths of accessibility to the_____ whenever possible.
    A. the bedroom, bathroom, and dining room
    B. the bathroom, drinking fountain, and bedroom
    C. the drinking fountain, bathroom, and telephone
    D. the telephone, bedroom, and bathroom

12. If an employer fails to accommodate the physical or mental limitations of a disabled employee, what is this known as?
    A. Discrimination
    B. Unequal employment
    C. Limited working environment
    D. All of the above

13. The 2019 Assisted Living State Regulatory Review regulations described which of the following?
    A. Maximum number of residents allowed per unit
    B. Square footage allowed per resident unit
    C. Sufficient sizing for the use of assistive devices such as wheelchairs and walkers
    D. All of the above

14. Newer assisted living facilities should be designed with travel distances from corridor to building exits no more than _____ and overall maximum travel distances should not exceed _____.
    A. 200 feet; 400 feet
    B. 150 feet; 300 feet
    C. 250 feet; 500 feet
    D. 100 feet; 200 feet

15. During an emergency or disaster evacuation, what can become a major problem for residents?
    A. Incontinence
    B. Self-isolation
    C. Lack of proper nutrition
    D. Unable to maintain self-hygiene

16. Once a building has been evacuated staff should
    A. evacuate to safety and account for all the residents
    B. not enter the building anymore
    C. wait until there are further instructions from emergency personnel
    D. if and when it is safe, carefully check the facility, including bathrooms, to make sure everyone has evacuated

17. As a best practice, administrators can benefit in fire safety by doing what?
    A. Installing smoke detectors
    B. Installing sprinkler systems
    C. Involving residents in safety trainings
    D. All of the above

18. What is the National Fire Protection Association's current main focus on?
    A. Standardizing fire sprinkler systems
    B. Develop and maintain over safety codes and standards
    C. Providing emergency response trainings
    D. Working with fire departments, insurance companies, unions, and trade organizations

19. Making social and environmental changes through gardens, pets, and the outside community is known as
    A. an Eden Alterative
    B. a Green House
    C. a medical model
    D. a cultural change

20. Studies have shown that residents in a(n) _____ model experienced improved functional status and quality of care compared to residents in a(n) _____ model.
    A. traditional; Green House
    B. Green House; traditional
    C. Eden Alternative; Green House
    D. traditional; Eden Alternative

21. Services offered at assisted living facilities are a way to promote what?
    A. Dignity
    B. Autonomy
    C. Quality of life
    D. All of the above

22. In the case study, the doctor's immediate prescription to treat DL's depression is an example of which of the following?
    A. An Eden Alternative
    B. The Green House model
    C. A medical model
    D. Culture change

23. Which of these statements are true regarding assisted living facilities practicing the traditional model of care?
    A. Residents have less control of their environment, schedules, and interactions
    B. Residents have more control of their environment, schedules, and interactions
    C. Residents have the freedom to participate in their own care planning
    D. It is an ideal approach to ensure proper care and well-being

24. What are the major challenges in implementing a Green House model?
    A. Finances and regulations
    B. Staffing and space
    C. Oversight and regulations
    D. Finances and maintenance

25. Which of the following is the easiest practice in terms of being in compliance with state regulations?
    A. An Eden Alternative
    B. The Green House model
    C. A medical model
    D. Culture change

26. Elements of the medical care model focuses on which type of approach?
    A. Education and prevention
    B. Physiological and psychological changes
    C. Disease and treatment
    D. Maintaining quality of life

27. What are the challenges of implementing the Eden Alternative?
    A. Finances and regulations
    B. Staffing and space
    C. Oversight and regulations
    D. Finances and maintenance

28. Who is the key staff member or members in a Green House community?
    A. Administrator because they are in charge of the daily operations and safety of everyone
    B. Activities director because they provide meaningful activities and entertainment
    C. Certified nursing assistants because they do the bulk of the work within the household, including cooking, cleaning, managing the household, and nurturing residents
    D. All of the above

29. Which best describes the philosophy of a Green House community?
    A. It emphasizes larger households to encourage socialization and maintaining relationships
    B. It focuses on quality-of-life outcomes and meaningful relationships
    C. It emphasizes smaller households to provide support and growth of residents and staff
    D. B and C
    E. A and B

30. The staff being able to hang meaningful photographs for DL, ask for her advice on bird feeders, and invite her to pet therapy visits is an example of which of the following?
    A. Eden Alternative
    B. Green House Model
    C. Culture change
    D. All of the above
    E. A and C

31. Culture change involves _____ nursing homes, and supports individualized resident care.
    A. deinstitutionalizing
    B. institutionalizing
    C. transforming
    D. rethinking practices

32. What makes the Eden Alternative unique?
    A. It placed emphasis on culture change and autonomy
    B. It introduced the use of music in care settings
    C. It introduced pets, plants, and children in care settings
    D. It improved care settings by creating smaller, intimate surroundings for residents and staff

33. A new resident just moved in and the staff took the time get to know his interests before setting up photographs of his family and friends to make him feel right at home. This is an example of which of the following?
    A. An Eden Alternative
    B. The Green House model
    C. A medical model
    D. Culture change

34. Creating small homes helps residents maintain their individuality, choice, privacy, and dignity. This is known as
    A. an Eden Alternative
    B. the Green House model
    C. a medical model
    D. culture change

35. A medical problem focus for service and delivery is known as
    A. the Eden Alterative
    B. the Green House model
    C. a medical model
    D. culture change

36. What is culture change?
    A. A focus on person-directed values and principles
    B. Core values related to dignity, respect, choice, and purpose
    C. Reformulating the meaning of aging
    D. A and B
    E. All of the above

37. Aging in place can provide which type of benefits?
    A. Dignity and physical, social, and emotional support
    B. Financial assistance
    C. Intellectual and spiritual wellness
    D. All of the above

38. Aging-in-place is a _____ model
    A. Consumer-Oriented
    B. medical
    C. cultural change
    D. universal design

39. Which universal design strategy can help someone with macular degeneration?
    A. Replacing traditional doorknobs with levers
    B. Installing grab bars
    C. Widening doorways and hallways
    D. Installing digital assistants such as Alexa or Google Home

40. Why is there a need for more improvements in designing settings?
    A. To stay relevant in today's market and charge competitively
    B. There is an increased population of older adults and people with disabilities currently living or planning to move to an assisted living
    C. To stay current with new trends and technologies
    D. To have options for incoming baby boomers

41. Referring to the case study, why was HD hesitant to move into an assisted living?
    A. He did not need the extra services
    B. He was in denial about his age and care needs
    C. He was giving up his independence and personal space
    D. He was unhappy with the services offered

42. Compared to the _____, residents aging in place are _____.
    A. medical model; inactive participants and consumers of healthcare services
    B. person-centered care; active participants and consumers of healthcare services
    C. Green House model; active participants and not consumers of healthcare services
    D. medical model; active participants and consumers of healthcare services

43. When designing an assisted living facility, light switches, faucets, and thermostats should be mounted _____.
    A. 36 inches
    B. 32 inches
    C. 9 to 52 inches above the floor
    D. 3 feet × 3 feet

44. Successful aging-in-place means that
    A. the rhythm of the day has been planned for all residents
    B. residents are encouraged not to participate in activities of daily living
    C. residents have similar service plans for efficiency and accuracy
    D. facilities adjust their service plans so residents have opportunities to be involved

45. Other than caregivers, who else greatly contributes to someone successfully aging-in-place?
    A. Volunteers
    B. Families
    C. Physicians
    D. All of the above
    E. None of the above

46. When designing an assisted living facility, clear pathways should be at least
    A. 36 inches
    B. 32 inches
    C. 9 to 52 inches above the floor
    D. 3 feet × 3 feet

47. Which universal design strategy can help someone who navigates with assistive mobility devices?
    A. Replacing traditional doorknobs with levers
    B. Installing grab bars
    C. Widening doorways and hallways
    D. Installing digital assistants such as Alexa or Google Home

48. What are some side effects of relocation?
    A. Isolation and depression
    B. Costs and loneliness
    C. Isolation and dependency
    D. None of the above

49. Universal designs involve elements that can be used by everyone regardless of abilities, such as which of the following?
    A. Door handles that don't require gripping or twisting
    B. Alarm systems that are audible and visible
    C. Storage space that's accessible to all heights
    D. All of the above
    E. A and C

50. Which universal design strategy can help someone with severe arthritis?
    A. Replacing traditional doorknobs with levers
    B. Installing grab bars
    C. Widening doorways and hallways
    D. Installing digital assistants such as Alexa or Google Home

51. When designing an assisted living facility, or a roll-in space, showers should be
    A. 36 inches
    B. 32 inches
    C. 9 to 52 inches above the floor
    D. 3 feet × 3 feet

52. PACE (Program of All Inclusive Care for the Elderly) provides which types of services?
    A. Podiatry
    B. Dentistry
    C. Optometry
    D. Physical therapy
    E. All of the above

53. Which are examples of instrumentals of activities of daily living?
    A. Providing assistance with eating, bathing, getting dressed, toileting, transferring, grooming, walking, and continence care
    B. Participating in adult day healthcare at a facility a couple of times a week
    C. Providing compassionate care for people in the last phases of incurable disease so that they may live as fully and comfortably as possible
    D. Providing meal preparation, house cleaning, medication management, and transportation
    E. All of the above

54. Which is a factor of federal bias toward nursing home care coverage? Select all that apply
    A. Coverage for skilled nursing care is mandatory under federal law
    B. Anyone who is financially and medically eligible will be covered for skilled nursing care
    C. Home- and community-based services are only an optional benefit
    D. The cost-neutrality requirements limit access to prospective consumers
    E. All of the above

55. When an aging individual cannot access the support and services needed to safely stay in their home, they stand to lose which of the following:
    A. Their physical home and possessions acquired over a lifetime
    B. Their independence
    C. Daily routine
    D. Easy access to family, friends, neighbors, church, and other community services
    E. All of the above

56. The highest level of care is provided in
    A. assisted living facilities
    B. skilled nursing facilities
    C. independent living facilities
    D. unlicensed board and care facilities
    E. All of the above

57. According to this chapter, the high turnover for in-home supportive services (personal care service) providers is attributed to
    A. geographic limitations
    B. low wages
    C. poor working conditions
    D. a lack of training
    E. All of the above

58. Which of the following companies is in charge of monitoring ethical issues on new applications from elderly?
    A. American Medical Association
    B. Consumer Department
    C. DHX (Digital Health eXcellence)
    D. Both A and C

59. Lyft, Uber, and taxis are examples of
    A. transportation
    B. transportation driving surrogacy
    C. car companies
    D. None of the above

60. What is the principal function of information and communication technology (ICT)?
    A. Entertainment
    B. Communication only
    C. Creation, manipulation, storage, and display of electrical data and information
    D. Research

61. Which is one of the uses for voice-activiated assistants?
    A. Inform of scheduled appointments
    B. Remind about medications
    C. Call for help in case of emergency
    D. None
    E. All of the above

62. When was the first personal digital assistant developed?
    A. 1990
    B. 1965
    C. 2001
    D. 1984

63. ICT is often referred to as _____.
    A. the future
    B. not effective
    C. innovative
    D. a "young-man's" game

64. Which of the following is <u>not</u> an example of eHealth, teleMed, and mHealth?
    A. Electronic health records
    B. Videoconferencing
    C. Text messages
    D. Robotic surgeries

65. Which sheets does the U.S. Department of Homeland Security provide to the elderly regarding security?
    A. Online Finance Security
    B. Information on Financial Security
    C. 10 Top Tips
    D. The older adult information sheet and Basic Tips and Advice sheet

RESIDENT CARE MANAGEMENT

1. Which of the following does not accurately describe issues in assisted living communities regarding lesbian, gay, bisexual, and transgender (LGBT) persons? Check all that apply.
   A. The current cohort of older LGBT persons spent much of their (early) adult years in an environment wherein they were labeled "sick" by their medical system, "immoral" by their churches, "illegal" by their government, and "unfit" by their military
   B. Attitudes and experiences persist even when formal labels may not, and this has pervasive implications both for LGBT persons in assisted living, and those with whom they share such spaces
   C. Fortunately due to progressive state laws, such as California's laws related to LGBT persons, facility staff in those states no longer need LGBT training
   D. The attitudes and behaviors of other residents can only be broadly managed and are sources of some significant anxiety for LGBT persons

2. _____ are more likely to live with family members or with family support than to live in institutional settings, and most of the family caregiving responsibilities reside with women.
   A. Hispanic Americans
   B. Asian Americans
   C. African Americans
   D. Native Americans
   E. Gays and lesbians

3. Which group has prior experience as caregivers for family and have concerns that they may not have family, friends, or children to care for them as they age?
   A. Hispanic Americans
   B. Asian Americans
   C. African Americans
   D. Native Americans
   E. Gays and lesbians

4. _____ believe women serve important roles in the preservation and transmission of culture and values; they are viewed as life givers, healers, and essential for the health of the community.
   A. Hispanic Americans
   B. Asian Americans
   C. African Americans
   D. Native Americans
   E. Gays and lesbians

5. One barrier for older_____ adults to receive care is that they are primary caregivers for children or grandchildren.
   A. Hispanic American
   B. Asian American
   C. African American
   D. Native American
   E. Gays and lesbian

6. Past discrimination, relocation, trauma, and oppression are all factors in _____ not seeking support.
   A. Hispanic Americans
   B. Asian Americans
   C. African Americans
   D. Native Americans
   E. Gays and lesbians

7. Within the many diverse Asian subgroups, _____ represent the largest number of individuals residing within this cultural group and account for about 30% of Asian elders.
   A. Chinese
   B. Japanese
   C. Filipinos
   D. Koreans

8. Women from _____ families have traditionally assumed roles that demonstrated respect for male dominance in family and cultural settings.
   A. Hispanic Americans
   B. Asian Americans
   C. African Americas
   D. Native Americans
   E. Gays and lesbians

9. Language barriers are creating a problem when it comes to the delivery of care for _____.
   A. Hispanic Americans
   B. Asian Americans
   C. African Americans
   D. Native Americans
   E. Gays and lesbians

10. _____ describes the connections between an individual's lifestyle and their cultural background.
    A. Culture
    B. Ethnicity
    C. Diversity
    D. Heritage consistency

11. _____ identified the fear of discrimination as a barrier to seeking health and social services.
    A. Hispanic Americans
    B. Asian Americans
    C. African Americans
    D. Native Americans
    E. Gays and lesbians

12. _____ remain the largest non-White group throughout the United States.
    A. Hispanic Americans
    B. Asian Americans
    C. African Americans
    D. Native Americans
    E. Gays and lesbians

13. Which group fears for their personal safety in an institutionalized setting such as assisted living or skilled nursing facilities?
    A. Hispanic Americans
    B. Asian Americans
    C. African Americans
    D. Native Americans
    E. Gays and lesbians

14. Which group expects the concept of filial piety, in which children are to provide respect, loyalty, and care for their elders?
    A. Mexicans
    B. Native Americans
    C. Chinese
    D. Gays and lesbians

15. Language, family values, and the role of elders in society are a barrier to _____ seeking support.
    A. Hispanic Americans
    B. Asian Americans
    C. African Americans
    D. Native Americans
    E. Gays and lesbians

16. Family caregiving in the _____ culture is encouraged and valued.
    A. Hispanic American
    B. Asian American
    C. African American
    D. Native American
    E. LGBT

17. Which group values spirituality, trustworthiness, and places importance value on the community as a whole and group success as opposed to individual successes?
    A. Hispanic Americans
    B. Asian Americans
    C. African Americans
    D. Native Americans
    E. Gays and lesbians

18. Which of the following accurately describes survey results regarding the issue of "disclosure" among the LGBT communities?
    A. A community sample of LGBT adults ranging in ages from 21 to over 90 years of age that approximately one third of midlife and older lesbians and gay men maintained some fear and anxiety about disclosing their sexual orientation
    B. Reports further show that gay men place more conditions on disclosure than lesbians
    C. Typically, between one quarter and one third of respondents do not disclose their sexual orientation
    D. A and C

19. Of the following, which is not true about sexual orientation?
    A. Sexual orientation refers to one's "enduring sexual attraction to male partners, female partners, or both"
    B. Heterosexuality refers to all possible sexuality attractions
    C. Homosexuality refers to same-sex attraction for men only (e.g., male to male, or "gay") , not for women (female to female, or "lesbian")
    D. Bisexuality refers to attraction to both sexes

20. Which of the following statements is most accurate regarding work of psychologist Henry Murray and anthropologist Clyde Kluckhohn (1948)?
    A. That there are no universal human characteristics that can be stereotyped but that there are shared characteristics and that the notion that there are unique characteristics based on what they saw as the inescapable is merely the power of their imagination
    B. That there are only universal human characteristics and that shared characteristics—described as "socio-cultural unit[s]"—is merely universal characteristics but in a tribal context
    C. That there are universal human characteristics; that there are shared characteristics—described as "socio-cultural unit[s]"—and that there are unique characteristics based on what they saw as the inescapable fact that each individual's particular modes of feeling, needing, and behaving are never duplicated by any other individual
    D. That there are universal human characteristics but no truly "shared experiences" and that there are unique characteristics based on what they saw as the inescapable fact that each individual's particular modes of feeling, needing, behaving are never duplicated by any other individual

21. For which group are elders thought to possess wisdom and knowledge from prior experiences and given elevated status in homes, churches, and communities?
    A. Hispanic Americans
    B. Asian Americans
    C. African Americans
    D. Native Americans
    E. Gays and lesbians

22. As outlined in the textbook, which of the following best describes <u>cisgender</u>?
    A. Having a gender identity that does not resemble the traditional expectations of the bio-logical sex of birth; one's internal gender identity thus does not conform to the cultural expectations of one's biological sex and gender presentation
    B. Having a gender identity that corresponds to the traditional expectations of the biological sex of birth; one's internal gender identity thus conforms to the cultural expectations of one's biological sex and gender presentation
    C. Having no gender identity and thus cannot correspond to the traditional expectations of the biological sex of birth
    D. Having a gender identity that corresponds to the traditional expectations of the biological sex of birth at first but then, later in life, changes one's internal gender identity thus not conforming to the cultural expectations of one's biological sex and gender presentation

23. Which of the following best describes the support network concerns for LGBT older adults?
    A. Relative to heterosexual cisgender women and men of comparable ages, LGBT older adults are (up to three times) <u>more</u> likely to live alone but, fortunately, due to the inten-tionality of LGBT relationships, are equally as likely to be partnered
    B. Relative to heterosexual cisgender women and men of comparable ages, LGBT older adults are equally likely to live alone but are up to one third <u>less</u> likely to be partnered
    C. Relative to heterosexual cisgender women and men of comparable ages, LGBT older adults are up to three times <u>more</u> likely to live alone and are up to one third <u>less</u> likely to be partnered
    D. Relative to heterosexual, cisgender women of comparable ages, LGBT older women are up to three times <u>more</u> likely to live alone and are up to one third <u>less</u> likely to be partnered, but, interestingly, studies have not shown the same disproportion for older gay males

24. Which of the following statements best describes the heteronormative pattern of support seeking (e.g., Cantor & Mayor, 1978):
    A. Care is both expected and, first, sought from close, personal friends because of more positive relationship; then, second, from immediate (i.e., biological) kin; and then, third, from more distant kin
    B. Care is both expected and first sought from immediate (i.e., biological) kin and then more distant kin, followed by "others" and formal services
    C. Care is both expected and first sought from professionals; then, second, close friends; third, immediate (i.e., biological) kin; and then, last, distant kin

25. Which one of the following best defines <u>transgender</u>?
    A. A term that characterizes those whose gender identities are congruent with those typi-cally associated with the biological sex assigned at birth
    B. An overarching term that characterizes those whose gender identities are consistently the same, even though it may or may not be consistent with those typically associated with the biological sex assigned at birth
    C. A very limed term used in narrowly defined situations that cannot be generally charac-terized using other definitions
    D. An overarching term that characterizes those whose gender identities are incongruent with those typically associated with the biological sex assigned at birth

26. What is the function of skin?
    A. Protects from trauma, microorganisms, and sun exposure
    B. Regulates body temperature
    C. Aids in touch and proprioception
    D. Works in the synthesis of vitamin D and prevents loss of body fluids
    E. All of the above

27. How does aging alter immune function?
    A. Overall decrease in immune responses, decreases in immunity through decreases in B cell, and increases in autoimmune responses to self
    B. Decreases in cellular immunity with impairment of immune system regulations
    C. Both A and B
    D. None of the above

28. Which of the following does not happen to arteries and veins as we age?
    A. Blood vessels stiffen and twist due to an increase in collagen and a decrease in elastin levels
    B. Typically there is an increase in pressure that can damage the blood vessels
    C. Veins thicken, become more dilated, and less elastic
    D. Veins return deoxygenated blood from the periphery of the body more efficiently due to the decrease in elasticity

29. What changes are seen in the brain and nerves as one ages?
    A. A decreased number of neurons and an increased accumulation of changes in brain tissues, including plaques
    B. An overall decrease in brain size and weight
    C. Decreased blood flow to the brain
    D. Increases in sleep disorders and insomnia
    E. Decreases in short-term memory
    F. All of the above

30. Which type of muscle accounts for the majority amount of muscle in the human body?
    A. Skeletal muscle
    B. Smooth muscle
    C. Cardiac muscle
    D. All of the above

31. What is the percentage for the number of fall injuries reported in the emergency room?
    A. 60%
    B. 55%
    C. 15%
    D. 75%

32. What dietary changes are best for elder who are overweight?
    A. A reduction in carbohydrates
    B. A reduction in fat
    C. A reduction in overall calories
    D. None of the above

33. What statement best describes the cardiovascular system?
    A. The cardiovascular system consists of the heart and vascular system and a series of arteries and veins that carry oxygen and nutrients from the heart to all body systems and remove carbon dioxide and waste
    B. The cardiovascular system consists of the heart and is only responsible for the removable of waste from the blood
    C. The cardiovascular system consists of the heart and muscular tissue throughout the body and is responsible for the transfer of nutrients throughout the body
    D. None of the above

34. Which is the correct list of types of depression?
    A. Minor, subthreshold, subclinical, and major depression
    B. Minor, subclinical, and major depression
    C. Subthreshold, mild depression, major depression, minor depression
    D. None of the above

35. How many types of joints do we have in the human body?
    A. 1 type
    B. 2 types
    C. 3 types
    D. 4 types

36. What factors influence sarcopenia?
    A. Hormonal changes
    B. Altered protein synthesis
    C. Nutritional factors
    D. A lack of physical exercise
    E. All of the above

37. Older adults who are experiencing moderate bone loss should supplement their diet with
    A. 100 mg of calcium per day
    B. 150 mg of calcium per day
    C. 1000 mg of calcium per day
    D. 1500 mg of calcium per day

38. Which of the following best describes the respiratory system?
    A. Mouth, nose, trachea, diaphragm, chest muscles, and lungs
    B. Mouth, Nose, trachea, abdominals, chest muscles, and lungs
    C. Nose, trachea, diaphragm, chest muscles, and lungs
    D. None of the above

39. What types of muscle does the human body have?
    A. Skeletal muscle
    B. Smooth muscle
    C. Cardiac muscle
    D. All of the above

40. What are the two top causes of chronic pain for aging adults?
    A. Cancer and arthritis
    B. Arthritis and diabetes
    C. Diabetes and cancer
    D. Cancer and stomach ulcers

41. What dietary changes are best for elders who have cardiovascular disease, hypertension, or diabetes?
    A. A reduction in carbohydrates
    B. A reduction in fat
    C. A reduction in overall calories
    D. None of the above

42. What factors predispose elders to fecal impactions?
    A. Age-related changes, poor nutrition, a lack of exercise, poor hydration, and a decrease in colonic transit time
    B. Age-related changes, poor nutrition, a lack of exercise, and poor hydration
    C. Age-related changes, poor nutrition, poor hydration, and a decrease in colonic transit time
    D. Age-related changes, poor hydration, and a decrease in colonic transit time

43. What are alveoli?
    A. Spongy air sacks located in the lung tissue
    B. Spongy tissue located along the trachea
    C. A collection of cancerous tissue that can affect the lungs
    D. None of the above

44. Physiologic issues associated with aging include
    A. nutrition and mobility
    B. fall prevention, sleep, and pain management
    C. mental well-being
    D. Both A and B
    E. Both B and C

45. Which professionals can assist with the assessment of alcohol and substance abuse?
    A. Physicians
    B. Nurses
    C. Social workers
    D. Alcohol abuse experts
    E. All of the above

46. What is considered a normal part of the aging process?
    A. Sensory changes
    B. Decrease in intellectual performance
    C. Increase in working memory
    D. None of the above

47. What changes in weight are seen in elders who have heavy alcohol use?
    A. No change in weight
    B. Weight loss
    C. Weight gain
    D. Rapid fluctuations in weight gain/loss

48. Delirium and seizures are commonly seen in elders that are withdrawing from _____.
    A. opioids
    B. caffeine
    C. alcohol
    D. nicotine

49. Hospitalization and/or medication is sometimes needed for
    A. major depression
    B. minor depression
    C. subthreshold depression
    D. All of the above

50. Which mental health problem can co-occur with early stages of dementia?
    A. Dementia
    B. Depression
    C. Anxiety
    D. Psychosis

51. Which online resources should be considered when dealing with an elder's depression?
    A. Online elder depression forums
    B. Online elder depression videos
    C. Webpages such as American Association of Retired Persons, the National Institute of Mental Health, and the National Institute on Aging
    D. All of the above

52. The CAGE questionnaire is used to assess _____
    A. anxiety
    B. depression
    C. alcohol dependency
    D. mood disorders

53. Men generally have a greater loss of brain volume in the _____ and _____.
    A. temporal lobe; frontal lobe
    B. occipital lobe; frontal lobe
    C. parietal lobes; frontal lobe
    D. All of the above

54. The American Psychiatric Association (2000) criteria for alcohol dependence required _____ out of the seven listed criteria in order to consider alcohol dependence.
    A. three or more
    B. two
    C. one or more
    D. four

55. Evaluation and treatment for elders with alcohol dependence and abuse should be conducted by
    A. the first individuals to notice the signs
    B. professionals with expertise in this area
    C. professionals with general expertise
    D. family members

56. How many items are on the Mini-Mental Status Examination (MMSE)?
    A. 8
    B. 15
    C. 11
    D. 21

57. When assessing an elder for dementia, it is important that their _____
    A. history with neurological problems, prior cognitive or memory problems, and prior acute and chronic medical problems are known
    B. history with prescription medication and recreational drug use is known
    C. history of medical problems, and dietary choices is known
    D. None of the above

58. What has psychological developmental theories revealed related to thinking and aging?
    A. As we age our thoughts generally become more negative
    B. As we age our thoughts generally become more positive
    C. As we age our thoughts generally remain stable
    D. As we age our thought generally increases in complexity

59. Which factors influence alcohol and substance abuse in elders?
    A. Chronic pain
    B. Self-treat depression
    C. Social changes
    D. All of the above

60. According to Dr. Pippa Hawley (2017), what are some barriers to accessing palliative care?
    A. A lack of resources to refer to
    B. A lack of knowledge of existing resources
    C. A misunderstanding of palliative care
    D. Restrictive specialist palliative care service program eligibility criteria
    E. All of the above

61. Which supplement has been noted to improve memory?
    A. Vitamin B12
    B. Ginkgo biloba
    C. Garlic extract
    D. Both A and B
    E. Both B and C

62. Alzheimer's disease is the _____-leading cause of death in the United States.
    A. third
    B. fourth
    C. fifth
    D. sixth

63. Staffing in assisted living units and memory care units mainly consist of the following:
    A. Med technicians
    B. Nurse practitioners
    C. Registered nurses (RNs), licensed vocational nurses (LVNs), and nursing assistants who may be certified (CNA)
    D. Doctors

64. As disease and other forms of dementia increase there is a need for
    A. more research to find a cure
    B. more legislators advocating for patient rights
    C. the creation of more services to assist those with these diseases as well as their family
    D. more home agencies

65. Assisted living administrators must have a comprehensive understanding of all the following except:
    A. State regulations
    B. How state regulations interface with federally mandated Medicare regulations
    C. Nationally required Joint Commission requirements
    D. The geriatric book for doctors

66. In the third or most severe stage of Alzheimer's disease, the elder experiences which of the following:
    A. Seizures and difficulty swallowing
    B. Incontinence and inability to recognize family members
    C. Contractures
    D. All of the above

67. The numbers of elders dealing with dementia are expected to increase _____ within the next 20 years.
    A. in the United States
    B. in developing countries
    C. nationally
    D. globally

68. The Joint Commission is defined as which of the following?
    A. A national accrediting agency
    B. A state regulatory agency
    C. A health department agency
    D. A surveyor agency

69. Current research is focused on achieving the following:
    A. Diagnosing, disease prevention, and drugs to treat all stages of Alzheimer's disease
    B. Managing incontinence and the severe stages of Alzheimer's disease
    C. A cure that will eliminate Alzheimer's disease completely
    D. An effective drug to slow cognitive decline

70. What are some factors that increase the chance of a person experiencing depression?
    A. Medical problems, life transitions
    B. Loss of a family member and friends
    C. Loss of support systems
    D. All of the above

71. When can hospice begin?
    A. At any point of the disease
    B. At the start of the disease as long as treatment is has began
    C. Once treatment of the disease is stopped
    D. None of the above

72. Which list best describes the issues that are taken into account by palliative care specialist?
    A. Physical, psychological, spiritual, caregiver support, practical needs
    B. Physical, economical, spiritual, family support, practical needs
    C. Physical, emotional, economical, spiritual, caregiver support practical needs
    D. None of the above

73. Which is the important factor to remember when planning a patient's physical aspect of care?
    A. The patient's goals for their care
    B. The desired disease management
    C. The patient's current medication
    D. All of the above

74. When did Kaiser Permanente begin its Palliative Care Program that received the leadership award by California Coalition for Compassionate Care?
    A. 2011
    B. 2001
    C. 2002
    D. 2004

75. How many prognosis months are needed in order to be eligible for hospice care?
    A. 3 months
    B. 4 months
    C. 5 months
    D. 6 months

76. Which is one important factor when discussing a patient's wishes?
    A. Ensure that the patient's wishes are properly documented and communicated
    B. Ensure that the patient's expectations are in line with reality
    C. Both A and B
    D. None of the above

77. What are some common physical symptoms that palliative care specialists manage?
    A. Pain
    B. Fatigue
    C. Loss of appetite
    D. Insomnia
    E. All of the above

78. Which hospital was given the leadership award by California Coalition for Compassionate Care?
   A. Kaiser Permanente
   B. UCSF Medical Center
   C. Stanford Health Care—Stanford Hospital
   D. Huntington Memorial Hospital

79. What is an IDT?
   A. Interdisciplinary team
   B. Inter-disorder team
   C. Inter-displacement team
   D. None of the above

80. Which individuals are usually included in an interdisciplinary team?
   A. Physician, hospice physician, nurses, and hospice aids
   B. Social workers and bereavement counselors
   C. Clergy and other spiritual counselors
   D. Volunteers and speech-language, physical, and occupational therapists
   E. All of the above

81. Where is the Nursing Home Bill of Rights applicable?
   A. The community
   B. Nursing homes and assisted living facilities
   C. All of the above
   D. None of the above

82. Community based palliative care is usually provided by _____
   A. palliative care specialists
   B. certified nursing assistants
   C. adult children
   D. neighbors

83. Medicare, Medicaid, and the Veterans Health Administration covers
   A. hospice care
   B. palliative care
   C. Both A and B
   D. None of the above

84. Which is one common expectation elders have when moving into an assisted living community?
   A. The assisted living community will provide them with all services advertised
   B. The assisted living community will adapt to their changing needs
   C. The assisted living community will ask them to relocate once their needs change
   D. All of the above

85. What phrase best describes hospice care?
   A. Focused on caring, not curing
   B. Focused on treatment
   C. Focused on physical improvement
   D. All of the above

86. Which of the following is considered to be confidential information?
    A. Information that identifies residents
    B. Health information to a resident
    C. All documentation related to the provision of healthcare services
    D. Any payment for healthcare
    E. All of the above

87. Which of the following best represents the requirements placed under the Patient Self-Determination Act of 1990? At the moment of entry residents are provided with
    A. maintaining written policies and procedures for all adults receiving medical services
    B. written information regarding the individual's right under state law to make decision regarding medical care
    C. ensuring compliance with state laws regarding advance directives
    D. providing staff and community education on issues concerning advance directives
    E. All of the above

88. The rights of assisted living facility residents to have religious liberties are guaranteed by
    A. state laws
    B. county laws
    C. each individual assisted living facility
    D. the U.S. Constitution

89. What is identified in the Nursing Home Residents' Bill of Rights (Code of Federal Regulation, Title 42, section 483.10)?
    A. The right of communication
    B. The right of medical care
    C. The right to manage financial affairs
    D. All of the above

90. In how many state ombudsman programs is the ombudsman model established?
    A. 50
    B. 45
    C. 53
    D. 43

91. Federal Regulations, title 42, section 483.10 states
    A. that long-term care residents have the right to self-determination and a dignified existence
    B. that long-term care residents have the right to access and communicate with others
    C. that long-term care residents have the right to access and communicate with others and with services both inside and outside of their facility
    D. All of the above

92. Who assumes a role in protecting the rights of residents?
    A. Ombudsman
    B. Nurses
    C. Geriatric specialist
    D. Social worker
    E. All of the above

93. How do state assisted living regulations address privacy?
    A. Physical plant requirements
    B. The square footage requirements for residents' rooms
    C. The maximum number of residents allowed per room and bathroom requirements
    D. All of the above

94. Which is covered under the right related to financial affairs?
    A. Right to secure possessions
    B. Manage their own financial affairs
    C. Not have to pay for services covered by Medicare or Medicaid
    D. All of the above

95. Which statement is true of most assisted living facility state regulations?
    A. There is a large difference on the way they are expressed through the states
    B. There are large similarities on the way they are expressed through the states
    C. Many states do not have assisted living facilities state regulations
    D. None of the above

96. How many Americans reside in assisted living communities?
    A. 810,000
    B. 812,000
    C. 832,000
    D. 850,000

97. The concept of capacity is based on a resident's ability to
    A. understand their right to make choices and the benefit and risk of specific treatments
    B. communicate with others about decisions
    C. remain stable over time and consistent in their values and beliefs
    D. All of the above

98. Which issue or issues is the ombudsmen program facing?
    A. State implementation differs, which affects data collection
    B. Obtaining data from long-term care and assisted living facilities
    C. Balancing data collection versus advocacy goals
    D. All of the above

99. What is required for the residents' bill of rights?
    A. It is required in all assisted living facilities
    B. It must be posted in locations where residents and other individuals are able to see
    C. It is accessible by employees
    D. All of the above

100. What statement best defines autonomy?
    A. Autonomy refers to the personal freedom to take control of one's life without interfering or infringing on the right of other individuals
    B. Autonomy refers to a person's ability to make any decision that they please
    C. Autonomy refers to a person's ability to make decisions without judgment
    D. None of the above

101. Which of the following is an example of a barrier seen when trying to implement palliative care programs in assisted living facilities?
    A. Regulations in some states do not permit retention of a resident who needs skilled nursing care
    B. Dying or terminally ill residents (or their families) request transfer to a nursing home or hospital
    C. If "risk of death" was not in the service contract, the facility could be liable for failure to respond appropriately
    D. All of the above

ANSWERS AND RATIONALES

The questions in this certification/licensure review reflect the knowledge and expertise of certified assisted living administrators who have experience writing questions for state-based certification and licensure exams. Although the book can be used as a standalone resource for exam preparation, the questions throughout this book have also been written according to the chapters presented in the textbook, *Assisted Living Administration and Management: Effective Practices and Model Programs in Elder Care, Second Edition*. At the end of each rationale, you will find the corresponding textbook chapter where you can find and review more information on the topic before sitting for an RC/AL certification or licensure exam.

CHAPTER 1: ORGANIZATIONAL MANAGEMENT

1. Answer: **E**
   Long-term care (LTC) has been defined "as an array of health care, personal care and social services generally provided over a sustained period, 90 days or more, to persons with chronic conditions and with functional limitations" (Wunderlich & Kohler, 2001 pp 27). The National Institute on Aging defines LTC as "a variety of services designed to meet a person's health or personal care needs during a short or long period of time." (*For more information on this topic, please see Chapter 1 in the textbook.*)

2. Answer: **A**
   As the "Baby Boomer" generation begins to age, the demand for LTC services is expected to increase. (*For more information on this topic, please see Chapter 1 in the textbook.*)

3. Answer: **E**
   Adult day care programs are a type of LTC that offers social interaction and meals from 1 to 5 days a week, depending on the program. Some adult care programs provide transportation to and from the care center. Activities often include exercises, games, trips, art, and music. Some adult care programs include medical services, such as help taking medications or checking blood pressure. (*For more information on this topic, please see Chapter 1 in the textbook.*)

4. Answer: **E**
   The population is aging, and the elderly population is growing older and living longer. The fastest growing age group in the country is 85 years and older. (*For more information on this topic, please see Chapter 1 in the textbook.*)

5. Answer: **E**

One effort to address quality problems was the establishment of the Assisted Living Workgroup (ALW). In 2003, the ALW issued a report with recommendations for improving quality in assisted living. Included in their recommendations were the following components:

- Introduction
- Definitions and core principals
- Accountability and oversight
- Affordability
- Direct care services
- Medication management
- Operations
- Resident rights
- Staffing (*For more information on this topic, please see Chapter 1 in the textbook.*)

6. Answer: **A**

The following are the main types of paid LTC providers: home care, adult day care, adult day healthcare, senior housing, assisted living/community-based residential care, skilled nursing facility/nursing home, and continuing care retirement community (CCRC). (*For more information on this topic, please see Chapter 1 in the textbook.*)

7. Answer: **B**

The Assisted Living Workgroup (2003) included the following recommendations regarding preadmission disclosure within the resident rights component of their report: (a) Preadmission disclosure for specialized programs of care, including the process for assessing residents and establishing individualized service plans; (b) preadmission disclosure on advance directives; and (c) preadmission disclosure on end-of-life care. (*For more information on this topic, please see Chapter 2 in the textbook.*)

8. Answer: **A**

In their report for the Centers for Disease Control and Prevention, Caffrey et al. (2012) noted that more than one half of all residents in assisted living communities were aged 85 and over. (*For more information on this topic, please see Chapter 1 in the textbook.*)

9. Answer: **E**

In their report for the Centers for Disease Control and Prevention, Caffrey et al. (2012) noted that the majority of residents living in residential care facilities in 2010 were non-Hispanic white and female; more than half of all residents were aged 85 and over; and nearly 2 in 10 residents were Medicaid beneficiaries. Furthermore, almost 4 in 10 residents received assistance with three or more ADLs, of which bathing and dressing were the most common. More than three fourths of residents have had at least 2 of the 10 most common chronic conditions; high blood pressure and dementias were the most prevalent. (*For more information on this topic, please see Chapter 1 in the textbook.*)

10. Answer: **B**

It is difficult to identify the exact beginnings of assisted living. Keren Brown Wilson (2007) explored the historical evolution of assisted living. She wrote,

To my knowledge, the first written use of the term (and my first such use of it) was in a 1985 proposal to the State of Oregon to fund a pilot study whereby the services for 20 nursing-home-level Medicaid recipients would be covered in a new residential setting. By 1988, assisted living was being used in presentations at professional meetings and in early trade publication articles. (*For more information on this topic, please see Chapter 1 in the textbook.*)

11. Answer: **C**

In a report to Congress, the U.S. Department of Health and Human Services and the U.S. Department of Labor (2003) noted that by 2050, the number of individuals using paid long-term care services in any setting (e.g., at home, residential care such as assisted living, or skilled nursing facilities) will likely double from the 13 million using services in 2000 to 27 million people. This estimate is influenced by growth in the population of older people in need of care. (*For more information on this topic, please see Chapter 1 in the textbook.*)

12. Answer: **C**

More than half of states reported changes between June 2018 and June 2019 that will affect assisted living communities. Specifically, 27 states and the District of Columbia reported changes to a variety of requirements, either to the licensing requirements or to other regulations that also apply to assisted living providers (e.g., nursing scope of practice or life safety). (*For more information on this topic, please see Chapter 2 in the textbook.*)

13. Answer: **B**

One effort to address quality problems was the establishment of the Assisted Living Workgroup (ALW). Formed at the request of the U.S. Senate Special Committee on Aging, the ALW was a national effort of approximately 50 organizations representing consumers, providers, LTC and healthcare professionals, and regulators. (*For more information on this topic, please see Chapter 1 in the textbook.*)

14. Answer: **E**

Assisted living is increasingly popular for many reasons. Concerns regarding nursing home quality, states' interests in containing LTC costs, as well as consumer demand have produced a dramatic growth in the industry. In Assisted living, personalized care and supervision can be provided outside of an institutionalized environment, with an emphasis of optimizing physical and psychological independence. (*For more information on this topic, please see Chapter 1 in the textbook.*)

15. Answer: **E**

There has never been a single nationally accepted definition of assisted living facility. In general, assisted living communities offer room and board with provisions for assistance with activities of daily living (ADLs) such as bathing, dressing, eating, grooming, continence, and eating. In addition, assistance with transportation, housekeeping, laundry, obtaining medical and social services, the supervision of medications, as well as other medical needs is often offered. (*For more information on this topic, please see Chapter 1 in the textbook.*)

16. Answer: **E**

    Today, the CEAL is a collaborative of the following nine organizations:

    ■ Alzheimer's Association

    ■ American Assisted Living Nurses Association

    ■ American Seniors Housing Association

    ■ Argentum

    ■ National Association of States United for Aging and Disability

    ■ The Society for Post-Acute and Long-Term Care Medicine

    ■ Leading Age

    ■ National Center for Assisted Living

    ■ Pioneer Network (*For more information on this topic, please see Chapter 1 in the textbook.*)

17. Answer: **E**

    Residents enter assisted living communities from a variety of places, including (a) the community, (b) other assisted living communities, (c) skilled nursing facilities, (d) nursing homes, and (e) hospitals. (*For more information on this topic, please see Chapter 1 in the textbook.*)

18. Answer: **C**

    The Assisted Living Workgroup (2003) included the following recommendations regarding resident rights in its report *Assuring Quality in Assisted Living: Guidelines for Federal and State Policy, State Regulations, and Operations, to the U.S. Senate Special Committee on Aging*: Within the boundaries set by law, residents have the right to the following:

    A. Be shown consideration and respect;

    B. Be treated with dignity;

    C. Exercise autonomy;

    D. Exercise civil and religious rights and liberties;

    E. Be free from chemical and physical restraints;

    F. Be free from physical, mental, fiduciary, sexual and verbal abuse, and neglect;

    G. Have free reciprocal communication with and access to the long-term care ombudsmen program;

    H. Voice concerns and complaints to the assisted living residence orally and in writing without reprisal;

    I. Review and obtain copies of their own records that the assisted living residence maintains;

    J. Receive and send mail promptly and unopened;

    K. Private unrestricted communication with others;

    L. Privacy for phone calls and right to access a phone;

    M. Privacy for couples and for visitors;

    N. Privacy in treatment and caring for personal needs;

    O. Manage their own financial affairs;

    P. Confidentiality concerning financial, medical and personal affairs;

    Q. Guide the development and implementation of their service plans;

    R. Participate in and appeal the discharge (move-out) planning process;

    S. Involve family members in making decisions about services;

    T. Arrange for third-party services at their own expense;

    U. Accept or refuse services;

    V. Choose their own physicians, dentists, pharmacists and other health professionals;
    W. Choose to execute advance directives;
    X. Exercise choice about end-of-life care;
    Y. Participate or refuse to participate in social, spiritual, or community activities;
    Z. Arise and retire at times of their own choosing;
   AA. Form and participate in resident councils;
   BB. Furnish their own rooms, and use and retain personal clothing and possessions;
   CC. Right to exercise choice and lifestyle as long as it does not interfere with other residents' rights;
   DD. Unrestricted contact with visitors and others as long as that does not infringe on other residents' rights;
   EE. Rights that one would enjoy in their own home, such as coming and going; and
   FF. Residents' family members have the right to form and participate in family councils. (*For more information on this topic, please see Chapter 2 in the textbook.*)

19. **Answer: E**
    Activities of daily living include bathing, dressing, eating, grooming, continence, and eating. (*For more information on this topic, please see Chapter 1 in the textbook.*)

20. **Answer: E**
    States often utilize specific criteria that determine whether a person can be admitted to or retained in an assisted living community. These include the general condition of the resident, health-related conditions, functional conditions, physical function, cognitive function, behavioral problems, and health needs that may require the need for nursing care. A primary purpose of regulating admission and retention is to ensure that providers are able to meet the needs of the population they serve. (*For more information on this topic, please see Chapter 2 in the textbook.*)

21. **Answer: E**
    The Assisted Living Workgroup (2003) included the following recommendations regarding the provider responsibility regarding resident rights in its report *Assuring Quality in Assisted Living: Guidelines for Federal and State Policy, State Regulations, and Operations,* to the U.S. Senate Special Committee on Aging:
    A. Promote an environment of civility, good manners, and mutual consideration by requiring staff, and encouraging residents, to speak to one another in a respectful manner;
    B. Provide all services for the resident or the resident's family that have been contracted for by the resident and the provider, as well as those services that are required by law;
    C. Obtain accurate information from residents that is sufficient to make an informed decision regarding admission and the services to be provided;
    D. Maintain an environment free of illegal weapons and drugs;
    E. Obtain notification from residents of any third-party services they are receiving, and to establish reasonable policies and procedures related to third-party services;
    F. Report information regarding resident welfare to state agencies or other authorities as required by law;
    G. Establish reasonable house rules in coordination with the resident council;
    H. Involve staff and other providers in the development of resident service plans;
    I. Maintain an environment that is free from physical, mental, fiduciary, sexual and verbal abuse, and neglect;

J. An assisted living residence may require that providers of third-party services ensure that they and their employees have passed criminal background checks, are free from communicable diseases, and are qualified to perform the duties they are hired to perform. (*For more information on this topic, please see Chapter 2 in the textbook.*)

22. Answer: **E**
The Assisted Living Workgroup (2003) included the following recommendations regarding resident rights in its report *Assuring Quality in Assisted Living: Guidelines for Federal and State Policy, State Regulations, and Operations*, to the U.S. Senate Special Committee on Aging: Within the boundaries set by law, residents have the right to be shown consideration and respect, to be treated with dignity, and much more. (*For more information on this topic, please see Chapter 2 in the textbook.*)

23. Answer: **D**
Assisted living employers have two general duties under OSHA: first, to furnish employees with employment (and a place of employment) that is free from recognized hazards likely to cause death or serious physical harm and, second, to comply with the detailed occupational safety and health standards promulgated under OSHA. (*For more information on this topic, please see Chapter 2 in the textbook.*)

24. Answer: **C**
Under the terms of the federal Nursing Home Reform Law, direct care staff must complete at least 75 hours of initial training under the supervision of a registered nurse with a minimum of 2 years' experience and at least 1 year nursing experience in LTC. (*For more information on this topic, please see Chapter 2 in the textbook.*)

25. Answer: **E**
The Fair Labor Standard Act of 1938 is the primary federal law setting minimum wage, overtime pay, equal pay, recordkeeping, and child labor standards for employers in the assisted living industry. (*For more information on this topic, please see Chapter 2 in the textbook.*)

26. Answer: **D**
Federal statues impact the operations of assisted living. Some examples are (a) Americans with Disabilities Act, (b) Civil Rights Act of 1991, (c) Rehabilitation Act of 1973, (d) Family and Medical Leave Act, (e) Fair Housing Amendments Act, (f) Fair Labor Standards Act (FLSA), and (g) Occupational Safety and Health Act. (*For more information on this topic, please see Chapter 2 in the textbook.*)

27. Answer: **A**
On average, 52% of people who turn 65 today will develop a severe disability that will require LTC at some point (Favreault & Dey, 2015). The average duration of need, over a lifetime, is about 2 years. While most people will need some LTC, only 14% are expected to need it for 5 years or more. (*For more information on this topic, please see Chapter 1 in the textbook.*)

28. Answer: **C**
To describe the various models relative to facility size and unit types, Zimmerman and Sloane (2007) describe a three-part typology to understand the multiple classifications of assisted living facilities across various states: (a) facilities with fewer than 16 beds, (b) larger homes

of the traditional board and care type, and (c) new model facilities with 16 beds or more—this new model facility is described as (a) built in or after 1987 and (b) having two or more private-pay rates, at least 20% of residents who required assistance in transfer, at least 25% of residents who were incontinent, or a registered nurse or licensed practical nurse on duty at all times. (*For more information on this topic, please see Chapter 2 in the textbook.*)

29. Answer: **A**
The Americans with Disabilities Act affects assisted living operators in two primary ways: first, as employers under Title I of that law and, second, as "public accommodations" under Title III of that law. (*For more information on this topic, please see Chapter 2 in the textbook.*)

30. Answer: **E**
For-profit investors want to see a profitable business that offers a safe, high return on their money. Investors want assurance that in your location, there's enough demand at the price you charge to make a good business. Furthermore, since for-profit investors want their money back, the business must either generate a lot of cash or be a good acquisition candidate. The aging of the population assures more and more people will be in need of LTC. (*For more information on this topic, please see Chapter 3 in the textbook.*)

31. Answer: **C**
More than half of the states and the District of Columbia report that provisions regarding assisted living concepts such as privacy, autonomy, and decision making are included in their assisted living regulations (Mollica et al., 2007). Overall, this philosophy represents a consumer-focused model in which the delivery of care is centered on the resident. (*For more information on this topic, please see Chapter 2 in the textbook.*)

32. Answer: **D**
The Green House Project continues to be one example of an innovative model of assisted living philosophy being adopted and integrated by assisted living communities across the nation. (*For more information on this topic, please see Chapter 3 in the textbook.*)

33. Answer: **A**
To understand the variation in state regulatory models, Carlson (2005) described two regulatory systems utilized by states: single level and multi level. In the single-level system, a state licensing agency licenses only one type of residential care/assisted living. In this model, any residential care/assisted living facility is licensed to accept or retain any resident, as long as the resident does not have a condition that disqualifies them from residential care/assisted living generally. In a multilevel system, residential care/assisted living facilities are licensed to care for residents only up to a particular care need. In this model, a resident typically may not be admitted or retained if they need a level of care that exceeds the specific level at which the facility is licensed. (*For more information on this topic, please see Chapter 2 in the textbook.*)

34. Answer: **D**
Assisted living facilities may sometimes cater to the specific needs of special populations. Examples include affiliations such as religious, ethnicity, or lesbian/gay/bisexual/transgender. (*For more information on this topic, please see Chapter 3 in the textbook.*)

35. Answer: **C**
Special care units (memory or dementia care) may promote a physical environment, activities, staff training, and program philosophy that address the special care needs of individuals

with memory loss and related behavioral problems. Activities such as art and music therapy are offered in units like these to aid with memory issues. Specialized dementia units often have a secure environment and a specialized physical design layout. (*For more information on this topic, please see Chapter 3 in the textbook.*)

36. Answer: **C**
    Small-group homes that provide care for seniors and frail elders have many names. Depending on location, they may be called board and care homes, assisted living, residential care homes for the elderly, personal care, adult foster care, adult group homes, adult family homes, or boarding care homes. (*For more information on this topic, please see Chapter 3 in the textbook.*)

37. Answer: **E**
    While both for-profit and not-for-profit assisted living communities accept resident rent as a source of an income, nonprofit organizations are also able to fundraise and accept donations. (*For more information on this topic, please see Chapter 3 in the textbook.*)

38. Answer: **E**
    To enhance the quality of life of persons with dementia, these specialty units will often include additional interventions and philosophies such as the following:
    - Holistic assessment
    - Regular formal assessments
    - Refer to other professionals as appropriate
    - Care planning involving resident, family, and staff
    - Provide person-centered care
    - Provide opportunities for residents to express themselves
    - Medication and nonpharmacological treatment
    - Training and management of staff
    - Provide positive and safe environment (*For more information on this topic, please see Chapter 3 in the textbook.*)

39. Answer: **C**
    There is no standardized service model in assisted living. There are advantages to this, such as flexibility for industry and consumers, wide variety of services (a community's option), and a wide range of structures (site-based and imported services, bundled and unbundled charges and services). There are also disadvantages to this variety. For example, there is less clarity. (*For more information on this topic, please see Chapter 3 in the textbook.*)

40. Answer: **E**
    Dating back to 1999, the U.S. Government Accounting Office (GAO) reported that most assisted living communities provide information about services offered but do not routinely provide information regarding discharge criteria, staff training and qualifications, services not available from the facility, grievance procedures, and medication policies. (*For more information on this topic, please see Chapter 2 in the textbook.*)

41. Answer: **E**

There are four common examples of different service models in assisted living, including the hospitality model, board and care, the specialized care model (i.e., dementia or memory care, and the larger scale model (also referred to as the newer model). (*For more information on this topic, please see Chapter 3 in the textbook.*)

42. Answer: **A**

Although very limited in availability, many (42) states now have several options for using Medicaid to fund services in assisted living communities (Carder et al., 2015). The majority of states currently utilize Home and Community Based Services waivers (also called 1915 (c) waivers) and others utilize state plans, while some utilize both. (*For more information on this topic, please see Chapter 2 in the textbook.*)

43. Answer: **E**

"Growing older without having to move" is frequently offered as a definition of *aging in place*. In comparison, the definition of aging in place offered by of M. Powell Lawton (1990) pp 287-288, a leader in aging research, described aging in place as a multidimensional phenomenon for seniors: "Aging in place represents a transaction between an aging individual and his or her residential environment that is characterized by changes in both person and environment over time with the physical location of the person's being the only constant." Catherine Lysack (2010) pp 620-621 expands on the idea that many elderly do not want to move as they get older: Baby boomers hope they can "live where they presently live until the end of life." (*For more information on this topic, please see Chapter 3 in the textbook.*)

44. Answer: **A**

Small-group homes that provide care for seniors and frail elders have many names. Depending on location, they may be called board-and care homes, assisted living, residential care homes for the elderly, personal care, adult foster care, adult group homes, adult family homes, or boarding care homes. These residences characteristically offer room and board in a small environment, typically housing 10 persons or fewer. These homes are commonly located in residential neighborhoods and offer a less institutional alternative. A homelike environment is of high priority. Because of the smaller number of residents, these homes often have very few staff. (*For more information on this topic, please see Chapter 3 in the textbook.*)

45. Answer: **D**

The administrator's objectives in both for-profit and nonprofit assisted living are the same: to meet the funding source's needs by laying out a plan for an organization that will get the job done better than other organizations. In for-profit, it's the bottom line that counts, and your community's plan will be geared around that. In nonprofits, it's what you do that matters, so you should set a business plan to meet that need. (*For more information on this topic, please see Chapter 3 in the textbook.*)

46. Answer: **E**

Aging in place is limited by several things in assisted living, including state regulation and community discretion. The models of care, regarding admission and retention criteria, discharge triggers, and the availability of hospice/end-of-life care, are all important to consider. (*For more information on this topic, please see Chapter 3 in the textbook.*)

47. Answer: **A**

The hospitality model in assisted living facilities offer apartment-style living and hotel-type services with limited personal care assistance. Services provided are meals, housekeeping, transportation, and security. Personal care services such as toileting, getting up from a chair, or assistance eating are limited. Residents have a high-degree of independence but may not be able to stay if their care needs worsen. (*For more information on this topic, please see Chapter 3 in the textbook.*)

48. Answer: **D**

Assisted living ideally allows the physical place to stay the same and implies that necessary services to meet an older person's needs be brought to them. Older persons usually move into supportive environments with the hope of avoiding other subsequent moves and that the community will be able to provide for their changing needs over time. The community's ability to do this is an important aspect of security for older people. (*For more information on this topic, please see Chapter 3 in the textbook.*)

49. Answer: **E**

The hospitality model in assisted living facilities may experience higher resident turnover rates, because of the lower level of care provided. Depending on size, this type of community will have varying number of staff. Hawes and colleagues (2000) classified an assisted living community to bear a low service status if it did not have an RN on staff and did not provide nursing care with its own staff. (*For more information on this topic, please see Chapter 3 in the textbook.*)

50. Answer: **E**

Although these "affiliated" communities do not discriminate against any person and still must comply with state regulations, they may offer services that are designed to benefit a distinct population for whom common values, language, food, and customs are promoted. (*For more information on this topic, please see Chapter 3 in the textbook.*)

51. Answer: **A**

In the report *High Service or High Privacy Assisted Living Facilities, Their Residents and Staff: Results From a National Survey* (2000), Hawes and colleagues made several conclusions regarding high-service assisted living facilities nationwide: (a) High-privacy or high-service assisted living facilities provide this care in a setting that has many components valued by consumers, particularly in terms of privacy and environmental autonomy; (b) most high-service or high-privacy assisted living facilities offered a wide array of services; (c) the issue of whether such services can meet residents' unscheduled needs is more complex; (d) the degree to which such facilities enable residents to age in place is clearly mixed unless one limits the concept to one of "*aging in place without significant decline in physical or cognitive functioning*"; and (e) assisted living is still a largely private-pay sector and, among the high-service or high-privacy assisted living facilities, one that is largely unaffordable for most moderate and low-income older persons unless they spend down their assets or receive help from relatives. (*For more information on this topic, please see Chapter 3 in the textbook.*)

CHAPTER 2: HUMAN RESOURCES MANAGEMENT

1. Answer: **D**
   Meadowlark Hills Retirement Community in Manhattan, Kansas, holds Learning Circles daily to address concerns and work through problems. (*For more information on this topic, please see Chapter 5 in the textbook.*)

2. Answer: **A**
   In Rhode Island, the Department of Health shall issue certification as an administrator for up to 2 years if the applicant is 18 years or older, of good moral character, and has initial training. (*For more information on this topic, please see Chapter 4 in the textbook.*)

3. Answer: **E**
   A successful interview is an effective interview. Characteristics of an effective interview include (a) providing information to the candidate about the facility, the agenda for the interview, and the job description; (b) being carefully planned and allow adequate time for each part of the process; (c) interviewers being prepared and information previously submitted by the candidate should be reviewed in advance of the interview; (d) carefully planned questions, developed in advance; (e) a core group of questions should be established that will be asked of all candidates; (f) the interviewer maintaining focus on the criteria for the position and the qualifications of the candidate; (g) the interviewer providing the candidate a realistic perspective of the job; (h) standards for performance and methods of evaluation being explained to the candidate; (i) providing the candidate with a description of employee benefits associated with the job; (j) a discussion of initial salary and salary ranges; (k) a description of the likely work schedule; (l) a tour of the facility; and (m) a follow-up letter regardless of if the candidate is hired or not. (*For more information on this topic, please see Chapter 4 in the textbook.*)

4. Answer: **B**
   Applicant screening involves the elimination of unqualified applicants from the recruitment pool. Screening every applicant to ensure a good fit is easiest to eliminate those with valid reasons for exclusion such as inadequate education or experience or failure to pass a criminal background check. (*For more information on this topic, please see Chapter 4 in the textbook.*)

5. Answer: **D**
   In New York, administrators generally must be at least 21 years of age, be of good moral character as evidenced by three letters of recommendations, and have varying levels of education and experience based in part on the number of residents in the facility. For example, in a facility with 24 beds or fewer, an administrator must (a) have a high school diploma or equivalency certificate, plus 3 years of related work experience, 1 year of which includes supervisory experience; (b) an associate degree from an accredited college or university in an approved course of study, plus 2 years of related work experience; or (c) a bachelor's degree from an accredited college or university in an approved course of study, plus 1 year of related supervisory work experience. The experience requirements increase as the size of the facility increases and are detailed in regulations. (*For more information on this topic, please see Chapter 4 in the textbook.*)

6. Answer: **D**

   Workforce recruitment in long-term care is often difficult because of the image of the indus-try. Ageism in society coupled with media reports of poor care quality, scandals, and elder abuse can bias the view of the public. Frontline worker jobs in long-term care are sometimes viewed by the public as unpleasant and poor paying. (*For more information on this topic, please see Chapter 4 in the textbook.*)

7. Answer: **C**

   Paraprofessionals (i.e., direct care staff) are those providing hands-on care directly to the residents in assisted living communities. They are by far the most important people in the organization and should be treated as such. This direct care staff are often referred to as the "eyes and ears" of the care system (Stone & Dawson, 2008). (*For more information on this topic, please see Chapter 6 in the textbook.*)

8. Answer: **B**

   The main components of the recruitment process are (a) planning, (b) searching, (c) screen-ing, (d) selection and hiring, and (e) maintaining applicant pool. (*For more information on this topic, please see Chapter 4 in the textbook.*)

9. Answer: **D**

   Some potential methods for recruiting candidates from external sources are community job fairs, advertisements in professional newsletters, community outreach programs, referrals from employees and friends, personnel placement service, and educational institutions. (*For more information on this topic, please see Chapter 4 in the textbook.*)

10. Answer: **B**

    The professional and paraprofessional workforce often lacks the necessary training to address the special health and medical care needs of the frail elderly. Adequate training is necessary to reduce high rates of staff injury and high rates of turnovers. (*For more information on this topic, please see Chapter 4 in the textbook.*)

11. Answer: **D**

    Projections or advanced knowledge of trends in the industry can assist in the planning of recruiting employees. It is important to consider the factors that influence workforce avail-ability (i.e., labor market and economy, wages and benefits, education and training, image of the industry, transportation). (*For more information on this topic, please see Chapter 4 in the textbook.*)

12. Answer: **B**

    Understanding unlawful questions and inquiries is critical to the interview process. Unlawful inquiries include, but are not limited to, questions about religion, age, childcare arrange-ments, and childbearing plans. (*For more information on this topic, please see Chapter 4 in the textbook.*)

13. Answer: **A**

    Planning recruitment efforts begins with forecasting employment needs. The assisted living administrator is responsible for projecting the needs (e.g., number of residents, levels of care) of the community and identifying the personnel requirements necessary to meet those needs. Advanced planning for employment needs are critical to the success of the community. (*For more information on this topic, please see Chapter 4 in the textbook.*)

14. Answer: **C**

    In Florida, administrators must complete 12 hours of continuing education every 2 years on topics related to assisted living. (*For more information on this topic, please see Chapter 4 in the textbook.*)

15. Answer: **E**

    Hiring and recruiting challenges are not entirely unique to a specific assisted living organizations—they are shaped by trends affecting long-term care employers across the country. This is especially true for paraprofessionals (i.e., direct care staff) due to low wages and benefits, hard working conditions, and work that is stigmatized by society. Furthermore, rarely do any of these workers receive adequate training to meet the demands of providing long-term care in a home setting, resulting in high rates of injury and high rates of turnover, reducing continuity of service. (*For more information on this topic, please see Chapter 4 in the textbook.*)

16. Answer: **A**

    In California, the law requires administrators, or facility managers and designated substitutes who may act on behalf of the administrator, must be at least 21 years of age. (*For more information on this topic, please see Chapter 4 in the textbook.*)

17. Answer: **C**

    Recruitment from individuals from within an organization can be beneficial for several reasons. Internal recruitment often allows for internal growth opportunities and may also result in greater retention, as well as improved staff morale and loyalty. Internal recruitment may be less expensive, less time-consuming, and less disruptive to a community. (*For more information on this topic, please see Chapter 4 in the textbook.*)

18. Answer: **A**

    Well-developed job descriptions are imperative to the planning phase of recruitment. Job descriptions are often utilized to establish salary ranges, define performance expectations, and evaluate performance, but they can also be very useful in a successful recruitment plan. (*For more information on this topic, please see Chapter 4 in the textbook.*)

19. Answer: **D**

    Justice in Aging identified five specific characteristics that should be considered when developing dementia training requirements. Those characteristics include (a) a comprehensive approach encompassing many settings and provider types and including managerial staff, (b) direct state involvement in development of training content and design of competency evaluations, (c) highly detailed training objectives, (d) outcome-based curriculum with examinations requiring a demonstration that competencies have been mastered, and (e) requirements for continuing education in addition to preservice training. (*For more information on this topic, please see Chapter 5 in the textbook.*)

20. Answer: **D**

    Justice in Aging, a national advocacy organization since 1972, identified Washington state as one state with strong and comprehensive models of dementia training requirements. Specifically, it identified five specific characteristics that should be considered when developing dementia training requirements. (*For more information on this topic, please see Chapter 5 in the textbook.*)

21. Answer: **C**

Learning circles are used in facilities nationwide and are changing the way management, staff, and residents communicate among one another. The purpose is to create an environment where people feel free to share their ideas and opinions without being criticized or reprimanded. This helps build trust among the participants which serves to strengthen relationships. Learning circles can be utilized in various ways, such as part of education and in-servicing. The learning circle is a leveling technique that encourages quiet people to speak, talkative people to listen, and everyone to share in making decisions. Participants observe, interpret, and experience not only their own feelings about an issue but also broaden their perspective by considering the many viewpoints around them. Learning circles are most effective when they become a way of life in the long-term care community and when everyone take a turn facilitating. (*For more information on this topic, please see Chapter 5 in the textbook.*)

22. Answer: **D**

The Assisted Living Workgroup (2003) provided the following recommendations based upon practice and research in long-term care facilities regarding orientation for all assisted living employees in its report *Assuring Quality in Assisted Living: Guidelines for Federal and State Policy, State Regulations, and Operations, to U.S. Senate Special Committee on Aging*:

Within 14 days of employment, all assisted living staff shall successfully complete an orientation program designed by the facility to provide information on the following:

1. The care philosophy of the assisted living facility.
    A. The understanding of dementia.
    B. The understanding of the common characteristics and conditions of the resident population served.
    C. Appropriate interaction with residents and family members.
    D. Customer service policies, including resident rights and recognizing and reporting of signs of abuse and neglect.
    E. Fire and life safety, emergency disaster plans, and emergency call systems.
    F. The use of facility equipment required for job performance.
    G. The facility's employment/human resource policies and procedures.

2. All staff shall have specific orientation relevant to their specific job assignments and responsibilities.

3. Contract staff should receive an orientation on topics relevant to their job tasks, including orientation of the facility's fire, life safety, emergency disaster plans, and emergency call systems. (*For more information on this topic, please see Chapter 5 in the textbook.*)

23. Answer: **C**

For decades, government agencies and advocates have identified undertrained staff in assisted living as a concern. The U.S. General Accounting Office (1999) identified insufficient and undertrained staff, low pay rates, and high staff turnover as major contributors to quality-of-care problems in residential care/assisted living. Carlson (2005) raised concerns regarding the experience and training of direct care staff. While state laws and regulations consistently require certain minimum training to be provided to direct care staff, the specifics of the training are often left to the individual communities. He cited numerous reports of the consequences of this inadequacy in training including incidence of staff failing to administer prescribed emergency medication for a diabetic, and failure of facility staff to recognize signs of acute infection resulting in the death of a resident (Carlson, 2005). In 2014, in an article written for the American Society on Aging, Patricia McGinnis wrote: "Few states devote adequate resources to enforcement and oversight of assisted living facilities, and nearly all states have inadequate staffing and staff training requirements." (*For more information on this topic, please see Chapter 5 in the textbook.*)

24. Answer: **C**
The Long-Term Care Community Coalition is a nonprofit organization dedicated to improving quality of care, quality of life, and dignity for elderly and disabled people in nursing homes, assisted living, and other residential setting. (*For more information on this topic, please see Chapter 5 in the textbook.*)

25. Answer: **E**
While some states specify only general requirements, others specify topics to be covered, the number of training hours required, the completion of approved courses, or some combination of topics, hours and courses. Common subjects in direct care staff training include recognizing and reporting elder and dependent adult abuse (including restraint use), general principles of assisted living, meeting the activities of daily living care/hygiene needs of residents, and meeting the needs of emotional and social needs of residents. (*For more information on this topic, please see Chapter 5 in the textbook.*)

26. Answer: **D**
Job descriptions are often utilized to establish salary ranges, define performance expectations, and evaluate performance, but they can also be very useful in a successful recruitment plan. Job descriptions contain detailed information on the skills, knowledge, abilities, and experience that a candidate should possess for a specific job. (*For more information on this topic, please see Chapter 4 in the textbook.*)

27. Answer: **E**
There are a variety of ways to recognize the value of each employee. Know your staff and call them by name. Let the staff see you daily on the unit and thank them for their work. Promote the value of the staff to all employees, residents, and families. Listen to the concerns of the staff. Involve staff with interview processes. Provide opportunity for crossover and shadowing in different departments. (*For more information on this topic, please see Chapter 6 in the textbook.*)

28. Answer: **A**
Peer review offers opportunities for growth. Encourage employees to participate in the development of standards for in-services, attendance, scheduling, routines, and policies. (*For more information on this topic, please see Chapter 6 in the textbook.*)

29. Answer: **D**
One way to recognize employees is the establishment of an "Employee of the Month" process in which those chosen are eligible for "Employee of the Year." Consider acknowledgment with a plaque, dinner, recognition in newsletters and monetary bonuses. This program must be well thought out. There should be internal guidelines on how it is run. (*For more information on this topic, please see Chapter 6 in the textbook.*)

30. Answer: **E**
The Paraprofessional Healthcare Institute a national organization, works to transform elder-care and disability services. It offers the following strategies for success growing a strong direct care workforce: (a) Recruit the Right Staff; (b) Improve the Hiring Process; (c) Strengthen Entry-Level Training; (d) Provide Employment Supports; (e) Promote Peer Support; (f) Ensure Effective Supervision; (g) Develop Advancement Opportunities; (h) Invite Participation; (i) Recognize and Reward Staff; and (j) Measure Progress. (*For more information on this topic, please see Chapter 4 in the textbook.*)

31. Answer: **F**
The administrator can create a positive work experience by establishing good working conditions. The administer must gain the respect of the employees and create an environment with positive morale. They must be consistent and reliable. There must be attendance policies and clear performance objectives. Supplies and equipment must be adequate. Training programs must be efficient. (*For more information on this topic, please see Chapter 6 in the textbook.*)

32. Answer: **E**
To understand the community's retention challenges, the administrator should review turnover, daily with all managers and department heads. All communities will experience turnover, but the extent of the turnover can be minimized with effective retention strategies. Turnover itself, depending on type, may be negative or positive. Warning signs that an employee is at risk for turnover include the employee (a) being visibly unhappy; (b) complains about workload or peers; (c) is experiencing life events, such as a divorce; (d) is using more sick time; (e) has unexplained absences; (f) has been rejected for a promotion or raise; (g) shows reduced interest in job; (h) exhibits a change in performance; and (i) loses peers or mentors who leave employment. (*For more information on this topic, please see Chapter 6 in the textbook.*)

33. Answer: **C**
To understand the community's retention challenges, the administrator should review turnover, daily with all managers and department heads. All communities will experience turnover, but the extent of the turnover can be minimized with effective retention strategies. Turnover itself, depending on type, may be negative or positive. (*For more information on this topic, please see Chapter 6 in the textbook.*)

34. Answer: **E**
Extrinsic factors associated with retention include (a) clean, safe work environments; (b) higher staff ratios; (c) union contracts for workers; (d) low rates of professional staff turnover; (e) positive relationships with residents, peers and supervisors; and (f) employee recognition. (*For more information on this topic, please see Chapter 6 in the textbook.*)

35. Answer: **A**
While many small associations have some local influence and offer continuing education, the larger organizations have a strategically planned advocacy program, often visiting lawmakers in their state capitals in large numbers to lobby for senior living. (*For more information on this topic, please see Chapter 7 in the textbook.*)

36. Answer: **A**
In a January 2019 publication, the Hospital and Healthcare Compensation Service reported that overall turnover in assisted living was down in 2018 as compared to 2017, but it was also up for some positions. Turnover across all positions declined from the 34.96% to 31.71%. Resident assistants and personal care aides turnover was 36.63% in 2017 and 33% in 2018, while dining service employee turnover increased from 35.74% to 36.91% in those same years. Improving retention rates is vital to improved quality outcomes in assisted living. (*For more information on this topic, please see Chapter 6 in the textbook.*)

37. Answer: **B**
Warning signs that an employee is at risk for turnover include the employee (a) being visibly unhappy; (b) complains about workload or peers; (c) is experiencing life events, such as a divorce; (d) is using more sick time; (e) has unexplained absences; (f) has been rejected for a promotion or raise; (g) shows reduced interest in job; (h) exhibits a change in performance; and (i) loses peers or mentors who leave employment. (*For more information on this topic, please see Chapter 6 in the textbook.*)

38. Answer: **D**
Gestures may go much further than monetary tokens. Never underestimate the power of saying "thank you." These gestures cost nothing and are personal and valuable. (*For more information on this topic, please see Chapter 6 in the textbook.*)

39. Answer: **E**
Extrinsic factors associated with turnover include (a) multiple employment opportunities, (b) inadequate job training, (c) excessive workload, (d) poor continuity of care, (e) a lack of respect, and (f) wages and benefits. (*For more information on this topic, please see Chapter 6 in the textbook.*)

40. Answer: **D**
Reward systems, when used strategically can promote staff retention and create positive working environments. Establish an internal committee comprised of managers and line-level staff from each department to assist in creating the recognition program. It should be multifaceted and be on an even playing field. Keep in mind that the goal is to reinforce quality and create coaching opportunities to boost performance. (*For more information on this topic, please see Chapter 6 in the textbook.*)

41. Answer: **E**
Some approaches to gaining important information from direct care staff include (a) requesting and accepting input from employees for changes to policies and procedures, (b) asking staff to share their problems and successes, and (c) seeking the participation of direct care staff in resident specific concerns. The administrator should not ask direct care staff to engage in duties beyond their job description or burden them with administrative/management duties. (*For more information on this topic, please see Chapter 6 in the textbook.*)

42. Answer: **A**
A staff recognition program is not optional; it is essential and the foundation of creating morale. Establish an internal committee composed of managers and line-level staff from each department to assist in creating the recognition program. (*For more information on this topic, please see Chapter 6 in the textbook.*)

43. Answer: **D**

Turnover refers to the number of staff that leave employment at the community for any rea-son. Retention means keeping valued employees. To understand the community's retention challenges, the administrator should review turnover, daily with all managers and depart-ment heads. The administrator's strategies should aim to minimize negative turnover and promote and maintain positive turnover. (*For more information on this topic, please see Chap-ter 6 in the textbook.*)

44. Answer: **F**

Hahklotubbe (2005) suggests that long-term care communities often overlook the concept of employee empowerment and hence are missing a key component of both employee pro-ductivity and job satisfaction. His research linked empowerment to morale and productivity in long-term care environments and identified employee empowerment as being frequently ignored as a way to potentially improve quality of care. Because job satisfaction is linked with retention, understanding and promoting employee empowerment is crucial for the assisted living community. There are some considerations that the administrator may take into ac-count in an effort to promote employee empowerment. (*For more information on this topic, please see Chapter 6 in the textbook.*)

45. Answer: **F**

Some additional, creative incentives to promote staff retention include (a) provide inexpen-sive vending items; (b) sponsor employee sports teams or purchase shirts printed with the community logo; (c) pay an allowance for uniforms, negotiate discounts for employees at local uniforms shops; (d) arrange for discounted purchases of bus passes; (e) provide free coffee or tea in the employee lounge; and (f) childcare support and assistance. (*For more in-formation on this topic, please see Chapter 6 in the textbook.*)

46. Answer: **E**

For those direct care staff providing care to residents with dementia, in addition to initial train-ing, they must receive an additional 8 hours annually. These include the following:

- Effects of medication on the behavior of residents with dementia
- Common problems such as wandering, aggression, and inappropriate sexual behavior
- Positive therapeutic interventions and activities such as exercise, sensory stimulation, activities of daily living, and social, recreational, and rehabilitative activities
- Communication skills and resident/staff relations
- Promoting resident dignity, independence, individuality, privacy, and choice
- End-of-life issues, including hospice (*For more information on this topic, please see Chapter 7 in the textbook.*)

47. Answer: **D**

Although the number of continuing education hours remained the same (i.e., 40 hours every 2 years), for administrators, the RCFE Reform Act specified minimum required knowledge for administrators in California:

- Knowledge of and ability to conform to the applicable laws, rules, and regulations
- Ability to maintain or supervise the maintenance of financial and other records (*For more information on this topic, please see Chapter 7 in the textbook.*)

48. Answer: **E**

There are a number of benefits to joining a professional association, including getting to know your local providers, gaining access to potential referral sources, and access to pipelines for staff recruitment. While all associations are unique in their agenda and purpose, some common threads are education, alliances, community service, member support, and networking. (*For more information on this topic, please see Chapter 7 in the textbook.*)

49. Answer: **D**

For those direct care staff providing care to residents with dementia, in addition to initial training, they must receive an additional 8 hours annually. (*For more information on this topic, please see Chapter 7 in the textbook.*)

50. Answer: **E**

Tim Clark (2013), Brand Contributor at Forbes explains the three generational workplace: Baby Boomers (a generation 76 million strong) are reaching the traditional retirement age, but many are continuing to work well into their 60s and 70s (and sometimes beyond). At the same time; Millennials (a generation 80 million strong) are advancing in their careers and beginning to take on leadership roles at their companies. Add in the Gen Xers (those in their mid-30s and 40s), and for the first time, we're seeing a workplace full of three generations (T. Clark, 2013). (*For more information on this topic, please see Chapter 7 in the textbook.*)

51. Answer: **C**

Gen Xers are those in their mid-30s and 40s. (*For more information on this topic, please see Chapter 7 in the textbook.*)

52. Answer: **D**

Stolee and colleagues (2005) found management support to "be the most important factor impacting the effectiveness of continuing education" (pp. 402). Administrators were acknowledged as the most instrumental person in long-term care, in terms of creating a better work environment that supports change. The study listed ways in which management could support continued education, like providing more funding for access to continuing education, and the required staff coverage. (*For more information on this topic, please see Chapter 7 in the textbook.*)

53. Answer: **D**

Millennials (a generation 80 million strong) are advancing in their careers and beginning to take on leadership roles at their companies. Furthermore, Millennials value engagement at work, which consists highly of training and personal development in their jobs. (*For more information on this topic, please see Chapter 7 in the textbook.*)

54. Answer: **B**

In response to several investigative reports about the failure in oversight and enforcement regarding assisted living communities in California, the RCFE (Residential Care Facility for the Elderly) Reform Act of 2014 was introduced (California Advocates for Nursing Home Reform, n.d.). The reform bills focused on improving care, empowering residents and providing the licensing agency with new tools to ensure compliance with regulatory standards. Specifically, legislative bill SB 911 (Block) expanded and specified continuing education requirements for staff in assisted living communities. (*For more information on this topic, please see Chapter 7 in the textbook.*)

55. Answer: **C**

The administrator plays a key role in ensuring that continuing education has a positive effect throughout the community. (*For more information on this topic, please see Chapter 7 in the textbook.*)

56. Answer: **F**

Healthcare system redesign is focused on system improvements, emphasizing teamwork, and health professions collaboration and communication (Brandt, 2015). (*For more information on this topic, please see Chapter 8 in the textbook.*)

57. Answer: **E**

Stolee and colleagues (2005) found that staff resistance to change, such as keeping their old ways and refusing change, was one of the factors hindering the effectiveness of continuing education in long-term care. (*For more information on this topic, please see Chapter 7 in the textbook.*)

58. Answer: **E**

In addition to the increased initial training direct care staff receive, direct care staff in California now must receive an additional 20 hours each year on specific topics:

- The aging process, physical limitations, and special needs of the elderly
- The importance and techniques of personal care services, including, but not limited to, bathing, grooming, dressing, feeding, toileting, and universal precautions
- Residents' rights and personal rights
- Medication policies and procedures
- Psychosocial needs of the elderly (e.g. recreation, companionship, independence, etc.)
- Recognizing the signs and symptoms of dementia in individuals
- Building and fire safety and appropriate response to emergencies
- Cultural competency and sensitivity in issues relating to the underserved aging LGBT community (*For more information on this topic, please see Chapter 7 in the textbook.*)

59. Answer: **D**

Attending conferences is an important aspect of continuing education for both administrators and direct care staff. Many conferences provide continuing education credits toward different certificates and licenses. In addition, conferences provide a networking opportunity for strong professional connections. (*For more information on this topic, please see Chapter 7 in the textbook.*)

60. Answer: **A**

Baby Boomers (a generation 76 million strong) are reaching the traditional retirement age, but many are continuing to work well into their 60s and 70s (and sometimes beyond). (*For more information on this topic, please see Chapter 7 in the textbook.*)

61. Answer: **E**

In response to several investigative reports about the failure in oversight and enforcement regarding assisted living communities in California, the RCFE Reform Act of 2014 was introduced (California Advocates for Nursing Home Reform, n.d.). The reform bills focused on improving care, empowering residents, and providing the licensing agency with new tools to ensure compliance with regulatory standards. (*For more information on this topic, please see Chapter 7 in the textbook.*)

62. Answer: **E**

    While there are many benefits to the latest technologies, such as ability to stop and start a course, learn at a specific pace, take the class in a native tongue, or go back and reinforce a concept, the argument that secondary gains of attending a classroom-style format are lost. These gains are having real-time questions answered by the facilitator or by a peer, real case examples of what is happening currently in other communities, and the ability to troubleshoot among professionals and peers a challenge you may be having in your community. Furthermore, there is value to expanding your network of other providers who may be a valuable resource in the future. (*For more information on this topic, please see Chapter 7 in the textbook.*)

63. Answer: **A**

    Despite the costs of healthcare delivery in the United States, patient outcomes remain worse in the United States than in many developing or developed countries (Josiah Macy Jr. Foundation, 2013). (*For more information on this topic, please see Chapter 8 in the textbook.*)

64. Answer: **A**

    Physicians are educated and licensed to provide medical care for elders (Mauk, 2018). (*For more information on this topic, please see Chapter 8 in the textbook.*)

65. Answer: **F**

    Interprofessional teams are composed of individuals from a number of disciplines who are qualified to work with elders. Professions represented in interprofessional teams include dietetics, pharmacy, social work, medicine, dentistry, nursing, physical therapy, and occupational therapy. (*For more information on this topic, please see Chapter 8 in the textbook.*)

66. Answer: **E**

    Dr. Cristina Flores (2005), in a California study, surveyed certified assisted living administrators to identify their perceived need for additional knowledge in specific areas of practice. Areas in which *moderate need for knowledge* was identified by most participants included the following:
    - Public policy for the aged
    - Death and dying
    - Hospice regulations
    - Dementia regulations
    - Meeting the cultural needs of residents
    - Biology of aging
    - Nutrition and aging
    - Healthcare and service
    - Pharmacology
    - Exercise physiology
    - Women's health and aging (*For more information on this topic, please see Chapter 7 in the textbook.*)

67. Answer: **A**

    The Patient Protection and Affordable Care Act created incentives for healthcare providers to improve quality and safety outcomes through the use of value-based care rather than care that is volume-based (Nester, 2016). (*For more information on this topic, please see Chapter 8 in the textbook.*)

68. Answer: **F**

A number of external forces are facilitating U.S. healthcare delivery, including quality improvement measures, patient safety measures, increasing need for care transition improvements, escalating healthcare costs, redesign of healthcare practice, and federal and state healthcare policy initiation (Brandt, 2015). (*For more information on this topic, please see Chapter 8 in the textbook.*)

69. Answer: **F**

The RN is responsible for the delegation of care and treatment recommendations to licensed vocational nurses and nursing assistants as well as direct supervision of licensed vocational nurses and nursing assistants. The RN additionally can provide oversight of medication administration and direct patient care delivery (Scope and Standards of Assisted Living Nursing Practice, 2006). (*For more information on this topic, please see Chapter 8 in the textbook.*)

70. Answer: **F**

Common elements of the chaplain role include assessment of eldercare plans, religious ritual and prayer facilitation, leadership within healthcare settings, ethical decision-making, and consultation and education for patients and staff members (Standards of Practice for Professional Chaplains in Long-term Care, 2012). (*For more information on this topic, please see Chapter 8 in the textbook.*)

71. Answer: **C**

The physical therapist role encompasses assessment of an individual's functional status and rehabilitation (Mauk, 2018). (*For more information on this topic, please see Chapter 8 in the textbook.*)

72. Answer: **C**

Mutual respect is an essential component of interprofessional practice (Nester, 2016). (*For more information on this topic, please see Chapter 8 in the textbook.*)

73. Answer: **E**

A lack of teamwork, inadequate communication, and limited collaboration were identified as responsible for many adverse health system and patient outcomes (Brandt, 2015). (*For more information on this topic, please see Chapter 8 in the textbook.*)

74. Answer: **B**

Poor communication has been linked to medical errors as well as quality and safety problems (Vega & Bernard, 2016). (*For more information on this topic, please see Chapter 8 in the textbook.*)

75. Answer: **A**

Oral health screenings were approved to address unmet oral health needs of elders in assisted living and long-term care settings (Romaszewski, 2017). (*For more information on this topic, please see Chapter 8 in the textbook.*)

76. Answer: **F**

Patient illness outcomes, staffing turnover, clinical error, mortality, and hospital readmission rates are decreased with the use of collaborative practice (Vega & Bernard, 2016). (*For more information on this topic, please see Chapter 8 in the textbook.*)

CHAPTER 3: BUSINESS AND FINANCIAL MANAGEMENT

1. Answer: **B**
   Assisted living communities face liability concerns whenever a medication mistake is made, particularly when residents are overdosed. If a resident is incapable of self-administration as defined within their state, the facility must be able to explain how the resident nonetheless continued to receive medication. (*For more information on this topic, please see Chapter 11 in the textbook.*)

2. Answer: **D**
   In its use in Japan, it is generally attributed four distinct process steps: (a) continuous improvement, (b) a belief in the process working, (c) understanding how the product is used, and (d) the process should have an aesthetic property. (*For more information on this topic, please see Chapter 9 in the textbook.*)

3. Answer: **B**
   The business plan should also be viewed as a strategic plan that at a minimum will include (a) the context and environment for the organization including competing services; (b) the purpose and goals of the organization and the services it will provide; (c) the resources required and how they will be used, including cash flow requirements, estimate income and expenses and source of income; (d) who is/will be served including a target population profile; (e) the time frame of the business plan and its components; (f) business strategies; (g) facility operation; and (h) an understanding of the consumer and their expectations. (*For more information on this topic, please see Chapter 9 in the textbook.*)

4. Answer: **C**
   The business plan should also be viewed as a strategic plan that at a minimum will include (a) the context and environment for the organization including competing services; (b) the purpose and goals of the organization and the services it will provide; (c) the resources required and how they will be used, including cash flow requirements, estimate income and expenses, and source of income; (d) who is/will be served including a target population profile; (e) the time frame of the business plan and its components; (f) business strategies; (g) facility operation; and (h) an understanding of the consumer and their expectations. (*For more information on this topic, please see Chapter 9 in the textbook.*)

5. Answer: **B**
   A review of the literature finds the term *systems* used repeatedly. The "systems" concept (Churchman, 1968; von Bertalanfy, 1968) is the principles selected to plan and review an assisted living community's organization and its business and operational plans. (*For more information on this topic, please see Chapter 9 in the textbook.*)

6. Answer: **E**
   Some control points are resource utilization and the budget, service program control, monitoring process, quality controls, and resident inputs. Inherent to management is providing leadership for the assisted living community and supporting leadership within the components of the organization. (*For more information on this topic, please see Chapter 9 in the textbook.*)

7. Answer: **E**
   Upon completion of an evaluation, an organization must decide how to utilize the information gathered to better its operation and assure quality. Whatever decision is made, any change must: (a) focus on service processes and their outcomes, (b) have an adaptive process

for the organization, (c) a basis for improvement, (d) provide ways to adapt to changing conditions or new knowledge, and (e) have a means to correct failure to meet goals and objectives, provision of less than optimal service, or improve its cost basis. *(For more information on this topic, please see Chapter 9 in the textbook)*

8. Answer: **C**

   The management approach must fit within the budgetary limitations of the assisted living community.

   An assisted living community may not afford this executive staffing level, yet management must still fulfill the functions through existing staff sharing responsibility for the functions. The management approach and methodology should fit the needs and services of the assisted living community as opposed to selecting a management methodology.

   It is important not only to define the assisted living community's goals, activities, components, and functions but also to describe how they are connected and reliant upon each other. *(For more information on this topic, please see Chapter 9 in the textbook.)*

9. Answer: **E**

   The assisted living community should have a program for evaluating marketing activity (Churchill, Jr., 1979). Is it meeting the goals of the business plan? Are the methods being used cost-effective? How do the methods being used compare with those of competitors? How will the information from the evaluation be used to improve marketing, and what parts of the evaluation should be provided to other parts of the organization. *(For more information on this topic, please see Chapter 9 in the textbook.)*

10. Answer: **B**

    The third element of a negligence claim is causation. The alleged injuries of the victim must have been caused, at least in part, by the breach of the duty of care that occurred. *(For more information on this topic, please see Chapter 11 in the textbook.)*

11. Answer: **C**

    PPBS was developed in the Department of Defense in the early 1960s to better manage resources relative to desired outputs. *(For more information on this topic, please see Chapter 9 in the textbook.)*

12. Answer: **E**

    Team building has become part of the participatory management landscape. The use of a team includes a broader range of inputs and talents to management, planning, operation, decision-making, and quality control. Team participation is aimed at consensus, but there are times to when a decision must be made and requires a determination of who will make it. *(For more information on this topic, please see Chapter 9 in the textbook.)*

13. Answer: **D**

    Items such as accrued income, accrued expenses, depreciation, expense accounting, revenues and deductions are NOT included. Cash basis is more popular because it is much simpler than accrual basis. For example, it does not demand as much bookkeeping records. *(For more information on this topic, please see Chapter 10 in the textbook.)*

14. Answer: **D**

    One major step in this growth was Theory X and Theory Y (McGregor, 1960) that stemmed from Maslow's (1943, 1954) "hierarchy of needs" (i.e., physiological need, safety needs, social needs, esteem needs, and self-actualization). Theory Z (Ouchi, 1982) has often been thought of as a blend of Theory X and Y yet having more in common with Theory Y. (*For more information on this topic, please see Chapter 9 in the textbook.*)

15. Answer: **A**
Management has been defined as "both science and art" (Buttaro, 1994). (*For more information on this topic, please see Chapter 9 in the textbook.*)

16. Answer: **C**
"Scientific management" stems from the work of Taylor (1911) and was developed in a period that reflected "reductionism" as a principle. (*For more information on this topic, please see Chapter 9 in the textbook.*)

17. Answer: **D**
The bureaucratic organizational form (March & Simon, 1958) was first described by the sociologist Weber (1947). It features clearly delimited functions by component elements with rigid boundaries, and well-defined tasks and lines of authority and reporting. A top-down chain of command is created with separation of an organization into functions and outputs. (*For more information on this topic, please see Chapter 9 in the textbook.*)

18. Answer: **C**
One example of an advantage to accrual basis is that because it requires a more detailed description of the revenues and expenses, it increases the chances of an exact measurement of net income and loss. (*For more information on this topic, please see Chapter 10 in the textbook.*)

19. Answer: **A**
A "tort" is committed any time a person or a business violates a basic expectation of a civil relationship. Examples of torts include battery, slander, and medical malpractice. Tort law is different from contract or criminal law. The key elements to tort law are (a) a civil wrong against a person or property and (b) prosecuted by the victim or their representative. Many torts are addressed by courts as "personal injury" lawsuits. (*For more information on this topic, please see Chapter 11 in the textbook.*)

20. Answer: **C**
Furthermore, the statement of expenses should be departmentalized, thus enabling senior management to determine the actual income and expense of each department for proper analysis of efficiency (utilization of resources), profits (either a profit center or loss center), and so on. (*For more information on this topic, please see Chapter 10 in the textbook.*)

21. Answer: **B**
The framework for producing quality is the Deming cycle (Deming & Walton, 1989): *plan, do, check, and act.* A set of 14 points was defined by Deming and became the hallmark of the worldwide application of the Deming concepts. (*For more information on this topic, please see Chapter 9 in the textbook.*)

22. Answer: **C**
Administration is the combination of support services needed to maintain the organization and its operation. Administrative services generally do not include direct client services, with the possible exception of support in the completion of forms needed to maintain residents' status at the facility. Administration serves as an arm of management to maintain the control and flow of resources, interaction with government and insurance agencies, banking services,

and internal control of personnel and budgeting issues. (*For more information on this topic, please see Chapter 9 in the textbook.*)

23. Answer: **A**

On one side of the dilemma is resident autonomy, allowing residents to make their own decisions regarding risk and benefits, and choosing when and how they would like to walk or ambulate. On the other side of the dilemma is resident safety, which suggests that facility staff have a duty to prevent residents from falling. Assisted living communities should carefully document its resident fall care plans and be sure to note residents' acceptance or refusal of recommended fall prevention techniques. (*For more information on this topic, please see Chapter 11 in the textbook.*)

24. Answer: **D**

The law does not require that falls be prevented; it rather expects reasonable measures will be undertaken to minimize them at all times. (*For more information on this topic, please see Chapter 11 in the textbook.*)

25. Answer: **C**

The four most important elements of a valid contract are
- offer and acceptance;
- consideration;
- capacity; and
- writing. (*For more information on this topic, please see Chapter 11 in the textbook.*)

26. Answer: **B**

Monetary remedies are focused on compensation and making a victim whole. The money that is awarded to the victim is intended to return the victim to the position they were in prior to the commission of the tort. (*For more information on this topic, please see Chapter 11 in the textbook.*)

27. Answer: **D**

Most states limit the grounds for legally evicting a resident. Some common reasons include the following:
- The resident's medical needs exceed what can be provided by the facility.
- The resident violates the terms of the admission agreement or other documented rules of the facility.
- The facility is closing. (*For more information on this topic, please see Chapter 11 in the textbook.*)

28. Answer: **C**

There must be some sort of information and statistical data relating to each department or aspect of the business. Accounting is the system that accumulates data of quantitative nature relating to the activities taking place in the communities. Senior management and the financial administrator must be able to utilize this information to make key and sound managerial decisions. Accounting is also the interpretation of the results of the data, involving not only accumulation but also the correct interpretation and then effective communication within the organization. (*For more information on this topic, please see Chapter 10 in the textbook.*)

29. Answer: **A**

The balance sheet is used to depict the entire financial operation of the communities in terms of its assets, liabilities, and capital (stockholder's equity) at a given period in time makes it more clear. At times, an assisted living community might have its total liabilities greater than its total assets. (*For more information on this topic, please see Chapter 10 in the textbook.*)

30. Answer: **A**

    Likert (1961, 1967) defined four types of management systems: (a) exploitive authoritative system—managers decide direction and make decisions based on an organizational hierarchy; (b) benevolent-authoritative system—similar to the exploitive authoritative system except a reward system is provided within the hierarchy, (c) consultive system—there is up and down communication within the hierarchy, but decisions are still hierarchical, and (d) participative (group) system—directions and decisions are made across the organization hierarchy, and there is a shared responsibility for the specific direction and actions taken. (*For more information on this topic, please see Chapter 9 in the textbook.*)

31. Answer: **B**

    The residential accounts receivable report (Table 10.8) checks the assisted living community's fiscal operations from the income perspective. (*For more information on this topic, please see Chapter 10 in the textbook.*)

CHAPTER 4: ENVIRONMENTAL MANAGEMENT

1. Answer: **D**

   State regulations cover the life safety of residents as well as the number of staff per shift and the provision of safety trainings for staff (National Center for Assisted Living, 2019). (*For more information on this topic, please see Chapter 12 in the textbook.*)

2. Answer: **A**

   The most current NFPA Life Safety Codes note that larger buildings require more fire protection and more built in fire protection (Kaspar, 2008). (*For more information on this topic, please see Chapter 12 in the textbook.*)

3. Answer: **B**

   Recovery following a disaster can be enhanced by talking about the disaster, sharing feelings, returning to daily routines, and focusing on personal needs such as sleep, nutrition, and use of medications (Shih et al., 2018). (*For more information on this topic, please see Chapter 12 in the textbook.*)

4. Answer: **C**

   Generators and emergency equipment should be readily available in the event of power outages (Cefalu, 2006). (*For more information on this topic, please see Chapter 12 in the textbook.*)

5. Answer: **C**

   Assisted living facility hallways must accommodate equipment including oxygen tanks, and must have a minimum of 60 inches of clearance (Kaspar, 2008). (*For more information on this topic, please see Chapter 12 in the textbook.*)

6. Answer: **A**

   Effective communication and plan accessibility are essential for successful emergency plan implementation (U.S. Department of Labor, n.d.). (*For more information on this topic, please see Chapter 12 in the textbook.*)

7. Answer: **B**

Close friends or roommates should be evacuated together to reduce anxiety and stress (Cefalu, 2006). (*For more information on this topic, please see Chapter 12 in the textbook.*)

8. Answer: **B**

Life Safety Codes are created by fire safety experts and regularly updated to reflect the current standards of fire safety professionals (Wolf, 2002). (*For more information on this topic, please see Chapter 12 in the textbook.*)

9. Answer: **A**

Ambulatory residents should be evacuated first during an emergency (Cefalu, 2006). (*For more information on this topic, please see Chapter 12 in the textbook.*)

10. Answer: **A**

All 50 states have adopted the use of I-Codes at either the state or local levels. (*For more information on this topic, please see Chapter 12 in the textbook.*)

11. Answer: **C**

Paths of travel should ensure access to bathrooms, drinking fountains, and telephones whenever possible to individuals with disabilities (Americans with Disabilities Act, 1990). (*For more information on this topic, please see Chapter 12 in the textbook.*)

12. Answer: **A**

Discrimination is defined in the Americans with Disabilities Act (2009) in part as denial of employment, failure to make reasonable accommodations for physical or mental limitations of disabled employees. (*For more information on this topic, please see Chapter 12 in the textbook.*)

13. Answer: **D**

The Assisted Living State Regulatory Review of 2019 (National Center for Assisted Living, 2019) describes a number of regulations including maximum number of residents per unit, the square footage of each resident unit and sufficient sizing of assistive devices, including wheelchairs and walkers. (*For more information on this topic, please see Chapter 12 in the textbook.*)

14. Answer: **D**

Travel distances from corridor to building exit should be no more than 100 feet, and overall maximum travel distances should not be more than 200 feet (Kaspar, 2008). (*For more information on this topic, please see Chapter 12 in the textbook.*)

15. Answer: **A**

Incontinence can be a major problem for residents during an emergency or disaster evacuation (Cefalu, 2006). (*For more information on this topic, please see Chapter 12 in the textbook.*)

16. Answer: **D**

Staff should be sure to check the facility following evacuation in an emergency to ensure everyone has evacuated (Cefalu, 2006) (*For more information on this topic, please see Chapter 12 in the textbook.*)

17. Answer: **D**
Best practices in fire safety include the installation of smoke detectors, sprinkler systems, and implementation of safety trainings for residents. (*For more information on this topic, please see Chapter 12 in the textbook.*)

18. Answer: **B**
The current work of the National Fire Protection Association involves the development and maintenance of over 300 fire safety codes and standards. (*For more information on this topic, please see Chapter 12 in the textbook.*)

19. Answer: **A**
The Eden Alternative involves the implementation of social and environmental changes through the use of gardens, pets, and the outside community (Rabig et al., 2006). (*For more information on this topic, please see Chapter 13 in the textbook.*)

20. Answer: **B**
Residents in facilities using the Green House model experienced improved functional status and quality of care compared to the traditional model (Rabig et al., 2006). (*For more information on this topic, please see Chapter 13 in the textbook.*)

21. Answer: **D**
The Assisted Living Workgroup (2003) report to the U.S. Senate Special Committee on Aging Topic Group recommendations reported on a philosophy to promote dignity, autonomy, and quality of life through assisted living facility services. (*For more information on this topic, please see Chapter 13 in the textbook.*)

22. Answer: **C**
The doctor's initial treatment of depression through medication prescription is an example of care in the Medical Model. (*For more information on this topic, please see Chapter 13 in the textbook.*)

23. Answer: **A**
Residents in assisted living facilities with traditional models of care have less control of their environment, schedules, and interactions. (*For more information on this topic, please see Chapter 13 in the textbook.*)

24. Answer: **A**
Implementation of finances and regulations are major challenges in implementation of the Green House model. (*For more information on this topic, please see Chapter 13 in the textbook.*)

25. Answer: **C**
The medical model allows for ease of practice in compliance with state regulations (National Center for Assisted Living, 2019). (*For more information on this topic, please see Chapter 13 in the textbook.*)

26. Answer: **C**
The medical care model is focused on disease and treatment. (*For more information on this topic, please see Chapter 13 in the textbook.*)

27. Answer: **D**

    Finances and regulations are the major challenges of implementation of the Eden Alternative. (*For more information on this topic, please see Chapter 13 in the textbook.*)

28. Answer: **C**

    Key staff members in Green House communities are certified nursing assistants performing the bulk of household work (Robert Wood Johnson Foundation, 2007). (*For more information on this topic, please see Chapter 13 in the textbook.*)

29. Answer: **D**

    The philosophy of a Green House Model community is focused on meaningful relationships, quality-of-life outcomes, and smaller households promoting resident and staff support and growth (Larsen, 2019). (*For more information on this topic, please see Chapter 13 in the textbook.*)

30. Answer: **E**

    The inclusion of pet therapy and the incorporation of advice on bird feeders and meaningful photographs occur within the Eden Alternative and cultural change. (*For more information on this topic, please see Chapter 13 in the textbook.*)

31. Answer: **A**

    Culture change involves a deinstitutionalization of nursing homes in support of individualized resident care (Pioneer Network, 2019). (*For more information on this topic, please see Chapter 13 in the textbook.*)

32. Answer: **C**

    The Eden Alternative is unique due to the introduction of pets, plants, and children in care settings (Burgess, 2015). (*For more information on this topic, please see Chapter 13 in the textbook.*)

33. Answer: **D**

    Culture change is focused on person-directed values allowing staff to determine resident interests upon entry into facilities (Pioneer Network, 2019). (*For more information on this topic, please see Chapter 13 in the textbook.*)

34. Answer: **B**

    The creation of small homes allows residents to maintain individuality, choice, privacy, and dignity in the Green House Model (Rabig et al., 2006). (*For more information on this topic, please see Chapter 13 in the textbook.*)

35. Answer: **C**

    A medical problem focus for service and delivery is known as the medical model. (*For more information on this topic, please see Chapter 13 in the textbook.*)

36. Answer: **E**

    Culture change is focused on person-directed values and principles, core values related to dignity, respect, purpose, choice, and a reformulation of the meaning of aging (Pioneer Network, 2019). (*For more information on this topic, please see Chapter 13 in the textbook.*)

37. Answer: **A**

Aging in place can provide individuals with dignity, physical, social, and emotional support. (*For more information on this topic, please see Chapter 14 in the textbook.*)

38. Answer: **A**

Aging in place is one example of a consumer-oriented model. (*For more information on this topic, please see Chapter 14 in the textbook.*)

39. Answer: **D**

The use of digital assistants such as Alexa or Google Home can provide a universal design strategy to help individuals with macular degeneration. (*For more information on this topic, please see Chapter 14 in the textbook.*)

40. Answer: **B**

An increased population of older adults and people with disabilities currently living or moving into assisted living have prompted a need for more design setting improvements (Vespa, 2018). (*For more information on this topic, please see Chapter 14 in the textbook.*)

41. Answer: **C**

In the case study, HD was hesitant to move into an assisted living facility because he would be giving up and losing his independence and personal space. (*For more information on this topic, please see Chapter 14 in the textbook.*)

42. Answer: **D**

Compared to the medical model, individuals aging in place are active participants and consumers of healthcare (Chapin & Dobbs-Kepper, 2001). (*For more information on this topic, please see Chapter 14 in the textbook.*)

43. Answer: **C**

When designing an assisted living facility, light switches, faucets, and thermostats should be mounted 9 to 52 inches above the floor (Mace et al., 1991). (*For more information on this topic, please see Chapter 14 in the textbook.*)

44. Answer: **D**

Successful aging in place means that facilities adjust service plans so residents have opportunities to be involved in care. (*For more information on this topic, please see Chapter 14 in the textbook.*)

45. Answer: **B**

Family members make significant contributions to successful aging-in-place strategies. (*For more information on this topic, please see Chapter 14 in the textbook.*)

46. Answer: **A**

Clear pathways in assisted living facilities should be at least 36 inches wide. (Mace et al., 1991). (*For more information on this topic, please see Chapter 14 in the textbook.*)

47. Answer: **C**

Widened doorways and hallways can provide a universal design strategy to help individuals using assistive mobility devices. (*For more information on this topic, please see Chapter 14 in the textbook.*)

48. Answer: **A**

Relocation frequently results in the side effects of isolation and depression for individuals relocating (Lawler, 2001). (*For more information on this topic, please see Chapter 14 in the textbook.*)

49. Answer: **D**

Elements of universal design that can be used by everyone include changes to door handles, alarm systems, and accessible storage spaces (Center for Inclusive Design and Environmental Access, 2012). (*For more information on this topic, please see Chapter 14 in the textbook.*)

50. Answer: **A**

The individual with severe arthritis can benefit from universal design replacing doorknobs with levers. (*For more information on this topic, please see Chapter 14 in the textbook.*)

51. Answer: **D**

Showers should be 3 feet × 3 feet when designing an assisted living facility (Mace et al., 1991). (*For more information on this topic, please see Chapter 14 in the textbook.*)

52. Answer: **E**

The program offers adult day healthcare at a PACE center, home health, meals at the center or delivered to the home, laundry services, physical and occupational therapy, and primary and specialty care, as well as preventative care such as audiology, podiatry, dentistry and optometry, case management, money management, durable medical equipment, prescription drugs, transportation, and socialization and recreation. (*For more information on this topic, please see Chapter 15 in the textbook.*)

53. Answer: **D**

Instrumental of activities of daily living such as bathing, dressing, meal preparation, shopping, laundry, and transportation to doctor's appointments. (*For more information on this topic, please see Chapter 15 in the textbook.*)

54. Answer: **E**

(a) Federal bias toward nursing home care. Coverage for skilled nursing care is mandatory under federal law. Anyone who is financially and medically eligible will be covered (Grabowski, 2006). (b) Home- and community-based services are only an optional benefit. Optional benefits lead to variation across the states and fragmentation within the states. (c) The cost-neutrality requirements limit access to prospective consumers (Newcomer et al., 2011). (d) There are no long longitudinal studies reporting the efficacy of the built in cost controls; therefore, it is difficult to measure the true value of diverting institutionalization. (*For more information on this topic, please see Chapter 15 in the textbook.*)

55. Answer: **E**

The transition out of their community into a facility can represent a loss of independence and the choice over their lifestyle and daily routine (Lecovich, 2014). A 2015 AARP study demonstrated the vast majority of people want to age in place, for reasons such as remaining in the community as long as possible to be close to family, friends, neighbors, church, and other community services (Barrett, 2014). (*For more information on this topic, please see Chapter 15 in the textbook.*)

56. Answer: **B**

    The highest level of care is provided in skilled nursing facilities. There are over 15,500 nursing homes nationally serving 1.3 million seniors and persons with disabilities. (*For more information on this topic, please see Chapter 15 in the textbook.*)

57. Answer: **E**

    The California Legislative Analyst Office (LAO) estimates that there is a 33% turnover rate for in-home supportive services workers, attributed to low home care wages and poor working conditions (Thomason & Bernhardt, 2017). High turnover resulting in unfulfilled care hours for the consumer causes adverse health effects and ultimately nursing facility placement if the recipient is unable to replace their provider (Thomason & Bernhardt, 2017). (*For more information on this topic, please see Chapter 15 in the textbook.*)

58. Answer: **D**

    To aid the ethical creation of applications for information and communication technology (ICT), the American Medical Association, American Heart Association, DHX (Digital Health eXcellence) Group, and Healthcare Information and Management Systems Society created and then implemented a cooperative guideline for consumers and developers alike in January 2018. (*For more information on this topic, please see Chapter 16 in the textbook.*)

59. Answer: **B**

    Today, depending upon how urban or rural the area, elders have several choices. If urban, taxi services or application transport companies (ATCs; Lyft™, Über™, etc.) are the easiest to arrange. (*For more information on this topic, please see Chapter 16 in the textbook.*)

60. Answer: **D**

    Information and communication technology is defined as information technology and other equipment systems, technologies, or processes, for which the principal function is the creation, manipulation, storage, display, receipt, or transmission of electrical data and information, as well as any associated content. (*For more information on this topic, please see Chapter 16 in the textbook.*)

61. Answer: **E**

    Some of the uses of voice-activated assistants (VAAs) will turn on certain televisions, play movies on command, and change the lighting in the room to set a mood or environment. VAAs can also tell your scheduled appointments, remind you of medications to take, and call for help in case of emergencies. (*For more information on this topic, please see Chapter 16 in the textbook.*)

62. Answer: **D**

    The first handheld uses of functional ICT were the personal digital assistant (PDA), and the self-contained power-source mobile telephone. The first PDA for the public (named the Organizer) was developed by Psion in 1984 and could only transfer input information onto a memory card that would then have to be downloaded into a computer for processing (Castelluccio, 2004). (*For more information on this topic, please see Chapter 16 in the textbook.*)

63. Answer: **D**

    Unfortunately, the creation of ICT for older adults today is a "young-man's" game. Many companies are doing research and development, testing and marketing of "elder care technology" without ever having had an "elder" see the product in development. (*For more information on this topic, please see Chapter 16 in the textbook.*)

64. Answer: **C**
In the United States, videoconferencing through use of home computers, smartphones, and tablets for medical purposes is becoming a trend. It has been conservatively estimated that at least 1 million doctor consultations were made by eHealth, teleMed, and mHealth in 2016 alone. Hospitals no longer "chart" on paper forms, and many surgeries are now done by robotic techniques. (*For more information on this topic, please see Chapter 16 in the textbook.*)

65. Answer: **D**
The U.S. Department of Homeland Security (2018a) has two fact sheets on how to arrest cybercrime, with one specifically created for older adults (2018b). The two fact sheets may seem very basic to a digital native, but for someone from the Baby Boomer generation or older, much of the tactics and or protection processes are of real value. (*For more information on this topic, please see Chapter 16 in the textbook.*)

CHAPTER 5: RESIDENT CARE MANAGEMENT

1. Answer: **C**
Notwithstanding California's progressive laws related to LGBT persons for facility staff training, the attitudes and behaviors of other residents can only be broadly managed—and are sources of some significant anxiety for LGBT persons (de Vries et al., 2019). (*For more information on this topic, please see Chapter 18 in the textbook.*)

2. Answer: **A**
Hispanic Americans are more likely to live with family members or with family support than living in institutional settings, and most family caregiving resides with women. (*For more information on this topic, please see Chapter 17 in the textbook.*)

3. Answer: **E**
Gays and lesbians have prior experiences as family caregivers and have concerns that they may not have care as they age. (*For more information on this topic, please see Chapter 17 in the textbook.*)

4. Answer: **D**
Native Americans believe that women serve important roles in the preservation and transmission of culture and values and are viewed as life givers, healers, and essential for community health (Walters et al., 2006). (*For more information on this topic, please see Chapter 17 in the textbook.*)

5. Answer: **C**
One barrier for older African American adults to receive care is that many serve as primary caregivers for children and grandchildren. (*For more information on this topic, please see Chapter 17 in the textbook.*)

6. Answer: **D**
Native Americans may not seek support due to past discrimination, relocation, trauma, and oppression. (*For more information on this topic, please see Chapter 17 in the textbook.*)

7. Answer: **A**
Chinese represent the largest number of individuals residing within Asian American cultural groups and account for about 30% of Asian elders. (*For more information on this topic, please see Chapter 17 in the textbook.*)

8. Answer: **B**
Women from Asian American families have traditionally assumed roles demonstrating respect for male dominance in family and cultural settings. (*For more information on this topic, please see Chapter 17 in the textbook.*)

9. Answer: **A**
Care delivery for Hispanic Americans can be problematic due to language barriers. (*For more information on this topic, please see Chapter 17 in the textbook.*)

10. Answer: **D**
Heritage consistency describes the connections between an individual's lifestyle and their cultural background. (*For more information on this topic, please see Chapter 17 in the textbook.*)

11. Answer: **E**
Gays and lesbians identified the fear of discrimination as a barrier to seeking health and social services. (*For more information on this topic, please see Chapter 17 in the textbook.*)

12. Answer: **C**
African Americans remain the largest non-White group throughout many areas of the United States (Agency for Healthcare Research and Quality, 2016). (*For more information on this topic, please see Chapter 17 in the textbook.*)

13. Answer: **E**
Gays and lesbians fear for their personal safety in institutional settings such as assisted living or skilled nursing facilities. (*For more information on this topic, please see Chapter 17 in the textbook.*)

14. Answer: **C**
The Confucian concept of filial piety is central in Chinese families, with children expected to provide respect, loyalty, and care for elders (Heying et al., 2006). (*For more information on this topic, please see Chapter 17 in the textbook.*)

15. Answer: **B**
Language, family values, and the role of elders in society can serve as barriers to Asian Americans seeking support. (*For more information on this topic, please see Chapter 17 in the textbook.*)

16. Answer: **C**
African Americans encourage and value family caregiving. (*For more information on this topic, please see Chapter 17 in the textbook.*)

17. Answer: **D**
Native Americans value spirituality, trustworthiness, and the community as a whole and value group success as opposed to individual successes. (*For more information on this topic, please see Chapter 17 in the textbook.*)

18. Answer: **D**

Research has often revealed that disclosure rates vary across groups and situations. Gardner et al. (2013) found, with a community sample of LGBT adults ranging in ages from 21 to over 90 years of age (and consistent with other research), that about one third of midlife and older lesbians and gay men maintained some fear and anxiety about disclosing their sexual orientation—this was particularly the case for lesbians, who also placed more conditions on disclosure (also noted in de Vries et al., 2019). (*For more information on this topic, please see Chapter 18 in the textbook.*)

19. Answer: **B**

Sexual orientation refers to one's "enduring sexual attraction to male partners, female partners, or both" (American Psychological Association, 2015). *Heterosexuality* refers to cross-sexuality attractions (e.g., male to female); *homosexuality* refers to same-sex attraction (e.g., male to male, or "gay"); female to female, or "lesbian")); *bisexuality* refers to attraction to both sexes (American Psychological Association, 2015). Recently, discussions of asexuality have appeared in the literature. (*For more information on this topic, please see Chapter 18 in the textbook.*)

20. Answer: **C**

More than 70 years ago, psychologist Henry Murray and anthropologist Clyde Kluckhohn (1948) wrote (paraphrasing the gendered language that was used) that in many respects, a person is (a) like all other people, (b) like some other people, or (c) like no other person. Murray and Cluckhohn were proposing the fundamentals of personality formation: the somewhat startling observation (at that time) that there are universal human characteristics (in a period of personality science when the focus of research was on what is unusual and distinguishing); that there are shared characteristics—described as "sociocultural unit[s]"; and that there are unique characteristics based on what they saw as the inescapable fact that each individual's particular modes of feeling, needing, and behaving are never duplicated by any other individual. This may be a useful and evocative framework for considering older adults and particularly older adults in assisted living communities. (*For more information on this topic, please see Chapter 18 in the textbook.*)

21. Answer: **C**

African American elders are thought to possess wisdom and knowledge from prior experience and are given elevated status in homes, churches, and communities. (*For more information on this topic, please see Chapter 17 in the textbook.*)

22. Answer: **B**

The question refers to the definition of cisgender as a gender identity corresponding to the traditional expectations of the biological sex of birth with one's internal gender identity conforming to cultural expectations of one's biological sex and gender presentations (American Psychological Association [APA], 2015). (*For more information on this topic, please see Chapter 18 in the textbook.*)

23. Answer: **C**

Relative to heterosexual, cisgender women and men of comparable ages, LGBT older adults are up to three times *more* likely to live alone and are up to one third *less* likely to be partnered (Adelman et al., 2006; MetLife Mature Market Institute, 2010; Wallace et al., 2011). (*For more information on this topic, please see Chapter 18 in the textbook.*)

24. Answer: **B**

    Much research reveals a heteronormative pattern of support seeking (e.g., Cantor & Mayor, 1978) wherein care is both expected and first sought from immediate (i.e., biological) kin and then more distant kin, followed by "others" and formal services. (*For more information on this topic, please see Chapter 18 in the textbook.*)

25. Answer: **D**

    Transgender is an overarching term that characterizes those whose gender identities are incongruent with those typically associated with the biological sex assigned at birth. (*For more information on this topic, please see Chapter 18 in the textbook.*)

26. Answer: **E**

    The skin regulates body temperature, aids in touch and proprioception, protects from trauma, microorganisms, and sun exposure and works in the synthesis of vitamin D to prevent loss of body fluids (Tabloski, 2006). (*For more information on this topic, please see Chapter 19 in the textbook.*)

27. Answer: **C**

    Aging alters immune function by decreases in immunity through decreased B cells and increases to autoimmune responses to self, as well as decreases in cellular immunity with impairment of immune system regulations (Tabloski, 2006). (*For more information on this topic, please see Chapter 19 in the textbook.*)

28. Answer: **D**

    As we age, veins do not become more efficient at returning deoxygenated blood from the periphery of the body due to decreases in elasticity (Mauk, 2018). (*For more information on this topic, please see Chapter 19 in the textbook.*)

29. Answer: **D**

    Changes to the brain and nerves seen with aging include decreased number of neurons, increased number of brain tissue changes including plaques, decreased blood flow to the brain, overall decrease in brain size and weight, increases in sleep disorders and insomnia, and decreases in short-term memory (Tabloski, 2006). (*For more information on this topic, please see Chapter 19 in the textbook.*)

30. Answer: **A**

    Skeletal muscles account for the majority of human body muscles. (*For more information on this topic, please see Chapter 19 in the textbook.*)

31. Answer: **A**

    The amount of fall injuries reported in the emergency room is 60%. (*For more information on this topic, please see Chapter 19 in the textbook.*)

32. Answer: **C**

    Overweight elders should reduce overall calories in the diet. (*For more information on this topic, please see Chapter 19 in the textbook.*)

33. Answer: **A**

    The cardiovascular system consists of the heart and vascular system, a series of arteries and veins that carry oxygen and nutrients from the heart to all body systems and remove carbon dioxide and waste. (*For more information on this topic, please see Chapter 19 in the textbook.*)

34. Answer: **A**

Minor, subthreshold, subclinical, and major are types of depression (Miller, 2009). (*For more information on this topic, please see Chapter 20 in the textbook.*)

35. Answer: **C**

There are three types of joints in the human body: immovable joints, cartilaginous joints, and synovial joints. (*For more information on this topic, please see Chapter 19 in the textbook.*)

36. Answer: **E**

Sarcopenia or reduction in muscle mass can be influenced by hormonal changes, altered protein synthesis, nutritional factors, or a lack of physical exercise (Mauk, 2018). (*For more information on this topic, please see Chapter 19 in the textbook.*)

37. Answer: **D**

Older adults with moderate bone loss should supplement with 1500 mg of calcium per day (Linton & Lach, 2007). (*For more information on this topic, please see Chapter 19 in the textbook.*)

38. Answer: **A**

The respiratory system consists of the mouth, nose, trachea, diaphragm, chest muscles, and lungs. (*For more information on this topic, please see Chapter 19 in the textbook.*)

39. Answer: **D**

The human body has skeletal, smooth, and cardiac muscles. (*For more information on this topic, please see Chapter 19 in the textbook.*)

40. Answer: **B**

The two major causes of chronic pain in aging are arthritis and diabetes (Miller, 2009). (*For more information on this topic, please see Chapter 19 in the textbook.*)

41. Answer: **B**

Elders with cardiovascular disease, hypertension, or diabetes should implement dietary changes reducing fat in the diet. (*For more information on this topic, please see Chapter 19 in the textbook.*)

42. Answer: **A**

Elders are predisposed to fecal impactions due to age related changes, poor nutrition, poor hydration, and a lack of exercise (Mauk, 2018). (*For more information on this topic, please see Chapter 19 in the textbook.*)

43. Answer: **A**

Alveoli are spongy air sacks located in the lung tissue. (*For more information on this topic, please see Chapter 19 in the textbook.*)

44. Answer: **D**

Physiologic issues associated with aging include nutrition, mobility, falls prevention, sleep, pain management, and mental well-being. (*For more information on this topic, please see Chapter 19 in the textbook.*)

45. Answer: **E**

Assessment of alcohol and substance abuse can be conducted by physicians, nurses, social workers, and alcohol abuse experts. (*For more information on this topic, please see Chapter 20 in the textbook.*)

46. Answer: **A**

Sensory changes occur as part of the normal aging process (Touhy & Jett, 2018). (*For more information on this topic, please see Chapter 20 in the textbook.*)

47. Answer: **B**

Elders who have heavy alcohol use may experience weight loss. (*For more information on this topic, please see Chapter 20 in the textbook.*)

48. Answer: **C**

Delirium and seizures are commonly seen in elders withdrawing from alcohol. (*For more information on this topic, please see Chapter 20 in the textbook.*)

49. Answer: **A**

Hospitalization and or medication may be needed to treat major depression (Miller, 2009). (*For more information on this topic, please see Chapter 20 in the textbook.*)

50. Answer: **B**

Depression can occur with early stages of dementia (Tabloski, 2006). (*For more information on this topic, please see Chapter 20 in the textbook.*)

51. Answer: **D**

A number of online resources should be considered when dealing with depression, including online elder depression forums, online elder depression videos, and webpages on depression. (*For more information on this topic, please see Chapter 20 in the textbook.*)

52. Answer: **C**

The CAGE questionnaire is used to identify alcohol dependency. The questionnaire is a self-reported four-question screening instrument (Mauk, 2018). (*For more information on this topic, please see Chapter 20 in the textbook.*)

53. Answer: **A**

Men generally have greater loss of brain volume than women do, especially in the temporal and frontal lobes (Tabloski, 2006). (*For more information on this topic, please see Chapter 20 in the textbook.*)

54. Answer: **A**

Three or more of the criteria for alcohol dependence identified by the American Psychiatric Association Committee on Nomenclature and Statistics (2000) are required to identify alcohol dependence. (*For more information on this topic, please see Chapter 20 in the textbook.*)

55. Answer: **B**

Evaluation and treatment for elders with alcohol dependence and abuse should be conducted by professionals with expertise in the fields of alcohol and substance abuse dependency. (*For more information on this topic, please see Chapter 20 in the textbook.*)

56. Answer: **C**

The Mini-Mental Status Examination contains 11 items (Touhy & Jett, 2018). (*For more information on this topic, please see Chapter 20 in the textbook.*)

57. Answer: **A**

When assessing elders for dementia, it is important to know any history of neurological problems, poor cognition, or memory problems and prior acute or chronic medical problems. (*For more information on this topic, please see Chapter 20 in the textbook.*)

58. Answer: **D**

Psychological developmental theories related to thinking and aging reveal that as we age our thoughts generally increase in complexity (Mariske & Margrette, 2006). (*For more information on this topic, please see Chapter 20 in the textbook.*)

59. Answer: **D**

Factors influencing alcohol and substance abuse in elders include chronic pain, social changes, and the use of these substances to self-treat depression (Touhy & Jett, 2018). (*For more information on this topic, please see Chapter 20 in the textbook.*)

60. Answer: **E**

Dr. Pippa Hawley (2017) wrote, "Despite significant advances in understanding the benefits of early integration of palliative care with disease management, many people living with a chronic life-threatening illness either do not receive any palliative care service or receive services only in the last phase of their illness" (abstract). Furthermore she identified some barriers to accessing palliative care:
   Lack of resources to refer to
   Not knowing that resources exist
   Ignorance regarding what palliative care is
   Reluctance to refer
   Reluctance of patient and/or family to be referred
   Restrictive specialist palliative care service program eligibility criteria (*For more information on this topic, please see Chapter 22 in the textbook.*)

61. Answer: **D**

Vitamin B12 and Ginkgo biloba have been noted to improve memory (Tablowsi, 2006). (*For more information on this topic, please see Chapter 20 in the textbook.*)

62. Answer: **D**

Alzheimer's disease is the sixth-leading cause of death in the United States. (*For more information on this topic, please see Chapter 21 in the textbook.*)

63. Answer: **C**

Staffing in assisted living units and memory care units mainly consists of registered nurses, licensed vocational nurses, and nursing assistants who may be certified (The Joint Commission (2014). Joint Commission Perspectives, 34(1), 8-13). (*For more information on this topic, please see Chapter 21 in the textbook.*)

64. Answer: **C**

As the rates of dementia increase, more services need to be created to assist those with dementia as well as the family members of dementia patients. (*For more information on this topic, please see Chapter 21 in the textbook.*)

65. **Answer: D**

    Assisted living administrators must have a comprehensive understanding of state regulations, the interface of state regulations with federally mandated Medicare regulations, and nationally required Joint Commission requirements. (*For more information on this topic, please see Chapter 21 in the textbook.*)

66. **Answer: D**

    The third or most severe stage of Alzheimer's disease is accompanied by seizures, difficulty swallowing, incontinence, contractures, and an inability to recognize family members (Alzheimer's Association, 2016; Mauk, 2018). (*For more information on this topic, please see Chapter 21 in the textbook.*)

67. **Answer: D**

    The numbers of elders dealing with dementia are expected to increase on a global level within the next 20 years. (*For more information on this topic, please see Chapter 21 in the textbook.*)

68. **Answer: A**

    The Joint Commission (2014) is a national accrediting agency established memory care unit requirements in 2014. (*For more information on this topic, please see Chapter 21 in the textbook.*)

69. **Answer: D**

    Current research is focused on identifying an effective drug to slow down cognitive decline. (*For more information on this topic, please see Chapter 21 in the textbook.*)

70. **Answer: D**

    Medical problems, life transitions, loss of family members or friends, and loss of support systems are some of the factors associated with depression in elders (Mauk, 2018). (*For more information on this topic, please see Chapter 20 in the textbook.*)

71. **Answer: C**

    Hospice care begins after treatment of the disease is stopped and when it is clear that the person is not going to survive the illness. (*For more information on this topic, please see Chapter 22 in the textbook.*)

72. **Answer: A**

    A palliative care specialist will consider the following issues for each person:

    Physical: Common physical symptoms include pain, fatigue, loss of appetite, weight loss, nausea, vomiting, shortness of breath, and insomnia.

    Psychological: Palliative care specialists can provide assistance to help persons and families deal with depression and anxiety related to their illness.

    Spiritual: Having to deal with a life-limiting and terminal illness, persons and families often look more deeply for meaning in their lives. Typically, one's illness brings them closer to their faith or spiritual beliefs, whereas others struggle to understand why it happened to them. Palliative care specialist can help people explore their beliefs and faith to help them find a sense of peace and bring them closer to accepting their situation.

    Caregiver Support: Family members are an important member of palliative care. Like the person, they have evolving needs. It is common for family members to feel overwhelmed by the heavy burden of responsibilities placed upon them. It is stressful trying to handle other duties, such as work, household tasks, and caring for other family members. Palliative care specialists can help families and friends cope and give them the support they need.

Practical needs: Palliative care specialists can also assist with financial and legal worries, insurance questions, and employment concerns. (*For more information on this topic, please see Chapter 22 in the textbook.*)

73. Answer: **A**

Physical care of seriously ill patients begins with an understanding of the patient goals in the context of their physical, functional, emotional, and spiritual well-being. The assessment and care plan focus on relieving symptoms and improving or maintaining functional status and quality of life. (*For more information on this topic, please see Chapter 22 in the textbook.*)

74. Answer: **D**

Kaiser's ideal program began in 2004 and continues to grow. Advanced healthcare planning is a primary focus, and many persons (including those living in assisted living communities) avoid hospitalization, transitioning to hospice when appropriate. (*For more information on this topic, please see Chapter 22 in the textbook.*)

75. Answer: **D**

The Medicare Hospice Benefit (n.d.) defines hospice eligibility as appropriate for patients when a doctor certifies a prognosis of 6 months to live and the person agrees to waive Medicare coverage for curative treatment. (*For more information on this topic, please see Chapter 22 in the textbook.*)

76. Answer: **A**

While more and more people are talking about end-of-life wishes, it is essential that those wishes are properly documented and communicated. This anticipatory guidance as included in the practice of a palliative care program can help keep people in place and ensure their wishes are being honored. The practice must be centered on the person's wishes and choices (J. Clark, 2003). (*For more information on this topic, please see Chapter 22 in the textbook.*)

77. Answer: **E**

A palliative care specialist will consider the following common, physical symptoms: pain, fatigue, loss of appetite, weight loss, nausea, vomiting, shortness of breath, and insomnia. (*For more information on this topic, please see Chapter 22 in the textbook.*)

78. Answer: **A**

One example of their successful programs is the Kaiser Permanente South San Francisco's Home Palliative Care Program. Its work was recognized in 2018 by the California Coalition for Compassionate Care with the leadership award (Wolfe, 2018). (*For more information on this topic, please see Chapter 22 in the textbook.*)

79. Answer: **A**

An expert panel of hospice professional develops a care plan that meets each person's individual needs for pain management and symptom control as called an interdisciplinary team (IDT). (*For more information on this topic, please see Chapter 22 in the textbook.*)

80. Answer: **E**
The interdisciplinary team usually consists of the person's physician, hospice physician, nurses, hospice aides, social workers, bereavement counselors, clergy or other spiritual counselors, trained volunteers, and speech, physical, and occupational therapists, as needed to provide comfort. (*For more information on this topic, please see Chapter 22 in the textbook.*)

81. Answer: **B**
The nursing home bill of rights is applicable in nursing homes and assisted living facilities (Code of Federal Regulations, Title 42, section 483.10). (*For more information on this topic, please see Chapter 23 in the textbook.*)

82. Answer: **A**
Palliative care is usually provided by palliative care specialists, healthcare practitioners who have received special training, and/or certification in palliative care. Often, palliative care specialists practice as part of an interdisciplinary team that may include doctors, nurses, registered dieticians, pharmacists, chaplains, psychologists, and social workers. (*For more information on this topic, please see Chapter 22 in the textbook.*)

83. Answer: **A**
Hospice care is covered by Medicare, Medicaid, the Veteran's Health Administration, and some private health insurance providers. Medicare and Medicaid cover hospice care for people with a terminal illness who meet admission criteria (both disease-specific criteria and a prognosis of 6 months or fewer) at no cost to the person, in most cases, while those who are covered by private health insurance plans may be responsible for copays and some other charges. (*For more information on this topic, please see Chapter 22 in the textbook.*)

84. Answer: **B**
When one decides on an assisted living community to move into, it is often their belief that they will be able to age in place, meaning that they expect the community will adapt to their changing needs so that relocation is not necessary. The key to aging in place is the community's ability to adjust the level of care to meet the resident's needs and avoid transfer to a higher level of care or skilled nursing facility. (*For more information on this topic, please see Chapter 22 in the textbook.*)

85. Answer: **A**
Considered the model program for quality compassionate care for people suffering from life-threatening illness, hospice care provides specialized medical care, pain management, and emotional and spiritual support expertly customized for individual person's needs and wishes, as well as the person's family. Hospice care focuses on caring, not curing. (*For more information on this topic, please see Chapter 22 in the textbook.*)

86. Answer: **E**
Confidential information includes information that identifies residents, health information, all documentation related to the provision of healthcare services, and any payment for healthcare (Tabloski, 2006). (*For more information on this topic, please see Chapter 23 in the textbook.*)

87. Answer: **E**

    The Patient Self Determination Act of 1990 details the responsibilities of healthcare providers to maintain written policies and procedures for all adults receiving medical services, provide written information regarding the individual's right under state law to make decisions regarding medical care, ensure compliance with state laws regarding advance directives, and provide staff and community education on issues concerning advance directives. (*For more information on this topic, please see Chapter 23 in the textbook.*)

88. Answer: **D**

    The U.S. Constitution guarantees the rights of assisted living facility residents to have religious liberties. (*For more information on this topic, please see Chapter 23 in the textbook.*)

89. Answer: **D**

    The Nursing Home Residents' Bill of Rights (Code of Federal Regulations, Title 42, section 483.10) identifies the following rights: the right to daily communication in one's language, the right to medical care, and the right to manage all financial affairs. (*For more information on this topic, please see Chapter 23 in the textbook.*)

90. Answer: **C**

    The ombudsman model is established in 53 state ombudsmen programs (Colello, 2008). (*For more information on this topic, please see Chapter 23 in the textbook.*)

91. Answer: **D**

    The Nursing Home Residents' Bill of Rights (Code of Federal Regulations, Title 42, section 483.10) notes the following rights: self-determination and a dignified existence, access to information and communication with others in the residents' own language, and access to services both within and outside of their facility. (*For more information on this topic, please see Chapter 23 in the textbook.*)

92. Answer: **E**

    Resident rights are protected by ombudsmen, nurses, geriatric specialists, and social workers. (*For more information on this topic, please see Chapter 23 in the textbook.*)

93. Answer: **D**

    State regulations of assisted living facilities address privacy issues for residents through physical plant requirements, resident room square footage requirements, bathroom requirements and the maximum number of residents allowed per room (National Center for Assisted Living, 2019). (*For more information on this topic, please see Chapter 23 in the textbook.*)

94. Answer: **D**

    The Nursing Home Residents' Bill of Rights (Code of Federal Regulations, Title 42, section 483.10) covers financial affairs including the rights to secure possessions, self-management of financial affairs, and non-payment for services covered by Medicare or Medicaid. (*For more information on this topic, please see Chapter 23 in the textbook.*)

95. Answer: **A**

    There is a large difference in the way assisted living facility state regulations are expressed throughout different states. (*For more information on this topic, please see Chapter 23 in the textbook.*)

96. Answer: **B**
There are 812,000 Americans residing in assisted living communities. (*For more information on this topic, please see Chapter 23 in the textbook.*)

97. Answer: **D**
The concept of capacity is based on a resident's ability to understand their right to make choices about the benefits and risks of specific treatments and to communicate with others about decisions. Capacity remains stable over time with consistency in the resident's values and beliefs (Miller, 2009). (*For more information on this topic, please see Chapter 23 in the textbook.*)

98. Answer: **D**
Issues faced by ombudsmen programs include different state implementation affecting data collection, data collection from long-term care and assisted living facilities is difficult, and the balancing of data collection with advocacy goals is also difficult (Netting et al., 1995). (*For more information on this topic, please see Chapter 23 in the textbook.*)

99. Answer: **D**
The Residents' Bill of Rights is required in all assisted living facilities and must be accessible to employees, and must be posted in locations where it can be viewed by residents and other individuals. (*For more information on this topic, please see Chapter 23 in the textbook.*)

100. Answer: **A**
Autonomy refers to the personal freedom to controlling one's life without interfering or infringing on the rights of other individuals (Miller, 2009). (*For more information on this topic, please see Chapter 23 in the textbook.*)

101. Answer: **D**
According to Mitty (2004), barriers to implementing palliative care programs in assisted living include:
Regulations in some states do not permit retention of a resident who needs skilled nursing care.
Dying or terminally ill residents (or their families) request transfer to a nursing home or hospital.
If the resident needs more care than was stipulated in the service contract, the resident cannot remain in the facility if additional services are needed for end-of-life care.
A nurse (RN or LPN) is not available on a 24-hour basis.
If "risk of death" was not in the service contract, the facility could be liable for failure to respond appropriately.
The assisted living residence is legally liable if a dying resident is not transferred to a nursing home or hospital unless the resident is a hospice patient.
There is insufficient reimbursement to the facility if it provides additional personal care.
The components, standards, or requirements of end-of-life care are unknown.
The facility has inadequate safe storage for pain management drugs.
Staff are uncomfortable being with a resident who is dying.
Physicians do not want their patients to die in an assisted living residence. (*For more information on this topic, please see Chapter 23 in the textbook.*)

REFERENCES

Adelman, M., Gurevitch, J., de Vries, B., & Blando, J. (2006). Openhouse: Community building and research in the LGBT aging population. In D. Kimmel, T. Rose, & S. David (Eds.), *Lesbian, gay, bisexual, and transgender aging: Research and clinical perspectives* (pp. 247–264). Columbia University Press.

Agency for Healthcare Research and Quality. (2016). *Chartbook on healthcare for Blacks.* https://www.ahrq.gov/research/findings/nhqrdr/chartbooks/blackhealth/index.html

Alzheimers's Association (2016) Alzheimer's disease facts and figures. Alzheimer's and Dementia, 12(4) 1–80. https:// doi.org/10.1016/j.jalz.2016.03.001

American Psychiatric Association. Committee on Nomenclature and Statistics. (2000). *Diagnostic and statistical manual of mental disorders* (4th ed., text revision).

Americans with Disabilities Act. (1990). http://www.doi.gov

American Psychological Association. (2015). *APA dictionary of psychology* (2nd ed.).

Assisted Living Workgroup. (2003). *Assuring quality in assisted living: Guidelines for federal and state policy, state regulations, and operations.* U.S. Government Printing Office. https://www.huduser.gov/portal/publications/Assuring-Quality-in-Assisted-Living-Guidelines.html

Alzheimers's Association. (2016). Alzheimer's disease facts and figures. Alzheimer's and Dementia, *12(4)*, 1–80. https://doi.org/10.1016/j.jalz.2016.03.001

Barrett, L. (2014). *Home and community preferences of the 45+ population 2014.* https://www.aarp.org/content/dam/aarp/research/surveys_statistics/il/2015/home-community-preferences.doi.10.26419%252Fres.00105.001.pdf

Brandt, B. F. (2015). Interprofessional education and collaborative practice: welcome to the "new" forty-year old field. *Advisor, 16*(1), 9–17. https://doi.org/10.3402/meo.v16i0.6035

Burgess, J. (2015). Improving dementia care with the Eden alternative. *Nursing Times, 111*(12), 24–25. http://www.nursingtimes.net/roles/older-people-nurses-roles/improving-dementia-care-with-the-eden-alternative-16-03-2015/

Buttaro, P. (1994). *Basic management for assisted living and residential care centers.* HCF Educational Service Publishers.

Caffrey, C., Sengupta, M., Park-Lee, E., Moss, A., Rosenoff, E., & Harris-Kojetin. (2012). *Residents living in residential care facilities: United States, 2010* (NCHS Data Brief, no. 91). National Center for Health Statistics. https://www.cdc.gov/nchs/data/databriefs/db91.pdf

California Advocates for Nursing Home Reform. (n.d.). *Introducing the RCFE Reform Act of 2014.* http://canhr.org/publications/newsletters/Advocate/FrontArticle/adv_2014Q1.htm

Cantor, M. H., & Mayer, M. (1978). Factors in differential utilization of services by urban elderly. *Journal of Gerontological Social Work, 1*(1), 47–61. https://doi.org/10.1300/J083V01N01_05

Carder, P., O'Keeffe, J., & O'Keeffe, C. (2015). *Compendium of residential care and assisted living regulations and policy: 2015 edition.* U.S. Department of Health and Human Services, Office of the Assistant Secretary for Planning and Evaluation, Office of Disability, Aging and Long-Term Care Policy and Research Triangle Institute. https://aspe.hhs.gov/basic-report/compendium-residential-care-and-assisted-living-regulations-and-policy-2015-edition

Carlson, E. (2005). *Critical issues in assisted living: Who's in, who's out and who's providing the care.* National Senior Citizen's Law Center.

Castelluccio, M. (2004). Writing on the screen. *Strategic Finance, 85*(11), 59–60.

Cefalu, C. A. (2006). Disaster preparedness for long-term care facilities. *Annals of Long-Term Care, 14*(9), 31–33 http://www.hmpgloballearningnetwork.com/site/altc/article/disaster-preparedness-long-term-care-facilities

Center for Inclusive Design and Environmental Access. (2012). *The goals of universal design.* www.universaldesign.com/what-is-ud

Chapin, R., & Dobbs-Kepper, D. (2001). Aging-in-place in assisted living. Philosophy versus policy. *The Gerontologist, 41*, 43–50. https://doi.org/10.1093/geront/41.1.43

Churchill, Jr., G. A. (1979). A paradigm for developing better measures of marketing constructs. *Journal of Marketing Research, 16*(1), 39–53. https://doi.org/10.1177/002224377901600110

Churchman, C. W. (1968). *The systems approach.* Delacorte Press.

Clark, J. (2003). Patient centered death. *BMJ, 327*(7408), 174–175. https://doi.org/10.1136/bmj.327.7408.174

Clark, T. (2013). *The 3-Generational Workplace: It's (Really!) A Good Thing.* https://www.forbes.com/sites/dailymuse/2013/12/02/the-3-generational-workplace-its-really-a-good-thing/#53c9259b965c

Colello, K. J. (2008). *Older Americans Act: Long-Term Care Ombudsman Program*. https://www.amazon
.com/OlderAmericans-Act-Long-Term-Ombudsman-ebook/dp/B005v5B285

de Vries, B., Gutman, G., Humble, A., Gahagan, J., Chamberland, L., Aubert, P., Fast, J., & Mock, S. (2019).
End-of-life preparations among LGBT older Canadians: The missing conversations. *International Journal
of Aging and Human Development, 88*(4), 358–379. https://doi.org/10.1177/0091415019836738

Deming, W. E., & Walton, M. (1989). *The Deming management method*. Dodd, Mead & Co.

Department of Homeland Security. (2018a). *Basic tips & advice*. Stop. Think. Connect. https://stopthink
connect.org/resources/preview/tip-sheet-basic-tips-and-advice

Department of Homeland Security. (2018b). Stop. Think. Connect. https://www.dhs.gov/sites/default/files/
publications/Cybersecurity%20for%20Older%20Americans_0.pdf

Favreault, M., & Dey, J. (2015). *Long-term services and supports for older Americans: Risks and financing
research brief*. U.S. Department of Health and Human Services. https://aspe.hhs.gov/basic-report/
long-term-services-and-supports-older-americans-risks-and-financing-research-brief

Flores, C. (2005). Assessing the needs of RCFE administrators. In D. Yee-Melichar & A. Boyle (Eds.), *Aging
in contemporary society: Translating research into practice* (pp. 17–25). XanEdu Publications.

Gardner, A., de Vries, B., & Mockus, D. (2013). Aging out in the desert: Disclosure, acceptance, and service
use among midlife and older lesbian and gay men in Riverside County. *Journal of Homosexuality, 61*(1),
129–144. https://doi.org/10.1080/00918369.2013.835240

Grabowski, D. C. (2006). The cost-effectiveness of non-institutional long-term care services: Review and
synthesis of the most recent evidence. *Medical Care Research and Review, 63*(1), 3–28. https://pdfs
.semanticscholar.org/e2c9/873a1fae819f695065c24361bc6abb044d4f.pdf

Hahklotubbe, D. (2005). Empowerment and long-term care: A contradiction in terms. In D. Yee-Melichar &
A. Boyle (Eds.), *Aging in contemporary society: Translating research into practice* (pp. 165–185). XanEdu
Publications.

Hawes, C., Phillips, C., & Rose, M. (2000). *High service or high privacy assisted living facilities, their residents
and staff: Results from a national survey*. Washington, DC: U.S. Department of Health and Human Services.

Hawley, P. (2017). Barriers to access to palliative care. *Palliative Care, 10*. https://doi.org/10.1177
/1178224216688887

Heying, J. Z., Guangya, L., & Guan, X. (2006). Willingness and availability: Explaining new attitudes toward
institutional elder care among Chinese elderly parents and their adult children. *Journal of Aging Studies,
20*(3), 279–290. https://doi.org/10.1016/j.jaging.2005.09.006

Josiah Macy Jr. Foundation. (2013, April 3). *Conference recommendations. Transforming Patient Care:
Aligning Interprofessional Education With Clinical Practice Redesign*. Josiah Macy Jr. Foundation. https://
macyfoundation.org/publications/aligning-interprofessional-education

Kaspar, J. (2008, February 1). *Protecting a vulnerable population*. http://www.csemag.com/articles/protecting
-a-vulnerable-population.org

Larsen, D. (2019). *The greenhouse project: The next big thing in long-term care*. Senior Living Blog. https://
aplaceformom.com/blog/green-house-project-next-big-thing-in-long-term-care

Lawler, K. (2001). *Aging-in-place. Coordinating housing and health care provision for America's growing
elderly population* (Report, Fellowship Program for Emerging Leaders in Community and Economic
Development).

Lawton, M. P. (1990) Knowledge resources and gaps in housing for the aged. In D. Tilson (Ed.), *Aging in
place: Supporting the frail elderly in residential environments*. 287–310. Scott, Foresman.

Lecovich, E. (2014). Aging in place: From theory to practice. *Anthropological Notebooks, 1*, 21–33 ISSN 1408-
032x Slovene Anthropoligical Society, 2014.

Likert, R. (1961). *New patterns of management*. McGraw Hill.

Likert, R. (1967). *The human organization: Its management and value*. McGraw Hill.

Linton, A. D., & Lach, H. W. (2007). *Concepts and practice. Gerontological nursing* (3rd ed.). Saunders Elsevier.

Lysack, C. (2010). Household and neighborhood safety, mobility. In P. Lichtenberg (Ed.), *Handbook of
assessment in clinical gerontology* (pp. 619–646). Elsevier.

Mace, R. L., Hardie, G. J., & Place, J. P. (1991) Accessible environments: Toward universal design. In
W. F. E. Pressler, J. Vischer, & E. T. White (Eds.), *Design interventions: Toward a more humane architecture*.
1–44. Van Nostrand Reinhold.

March, J., & Simon, H. (1958). *Organizations*. John Wiley.

Mariske, M., & Margrett, J. A. (2006). Everyday problem solving and decision making. In J. E. Birrin & K. W.
Schaie (Eds.), *Handbook of the psychology of aging* (6th ed., pp. 57–83). Academic Press.

Maslow, A. (1943). A theory of human motivation. *Psychological Review, 50*(4), 370–396. https://www
.academia.edu/9415670/A_Theory_of_Human_Motivation_Abraham_H_Maslow_Psychological
_Review_Vol_50_No_4_July_1943

Maslow, A. (1954). *Motivation and personality*. Harper & Row.

Mauk, K. (2018). *Gerontoligical nursing: Competencies for care* (4th ed.). Jones & Bartlett Learning.

McGregor, D. (1960). *The human side of the enterprise*. McGraw Hill.

McGinnis, Patricia. (2014). Assisted living: A crisis in care. American Society on Aging: Aging Today.
Retrieved October 22, 2019 from https://www.asaging.org/blog/assisted-living-crisis-care

Medicare Hospice Benefit. (n.d.). *Medicare hospice benefit definition*. https://www.medicare.gov/pubs/
pdf/02154-medicare-hospice-benefits.pdf

MetLife Mature Market Institute. (2010). *Still out, still aging*. MetLife Mature Market Institute.

Miller, C. A. (2009). *Nursing for wellness in older adults* (5th ed.). Lippincott, Williams, & Wilkins.

Mitty, E. (2004). Assisted living: Aging in place and palliative care. *Geriatric Nursing, 25*, 149–163. https://
doi.org/10.1016/j.gerinurse.2004.04.019

Mollica, R., Sims-Kastelein, K., & O'Keeffe, J. (2007). *Residential care and assisted living compendium, 2007*. U.S. Department of Health and Human Services, Office of the Assistant Secretary for Planning and Evaluation, Office of Disability, Aging and Long-Term Care Policy and Research Triangle Institute. https://aspe.hhs.gov/system/files/pdf/75316/07alcom.pdf

Murray, H. A., & Kluckhohn, C. (Eds.). (1948). *Personality in nature, society, and culture*. Alfred A. Knopf.

National Center for Assisted Living. (2019). *2019 Assisted living state regulatory review*. https://www
.ahcancal.org/ncal/advocacy/regs/Documents/2019_reg_review.pdf

Nester, J. (2016). The importance of interprofessional practice and education in the era of accountable care. *North Carolina Medical Journal, 77*(2), 128–132. https://doi.org/10.18043/ncm.77.2.128

Netting, E. F., Huber, R., Paton, R. N., & Kautz III, J. R. (1995). Elder rights and the long-term care ombudsman program. *Social Work, 40*(3), 351–357. https:// doi.org/10.18043/ncm.77.2.128

Newcomer, R., Harrington, C., Stone, J., Bindman, A. B., & Helmar, M. (2011). *California's Medi-Cal Home & Community-Based Services waivers, benefits & eligibility policies*, 2005–2008. University of California, San Francisco & California Department of Health Care Services. http://www.thescanfoundation.org/sites/
default/files/camri_waiver_report_0_3.pdf

Ouchi, W. G. (1982). *Theory Z*. Avon Books.

Pioneer Network. (2019). *Defining culture change*. https://www.pioneernetwork.net/culture-change/
what-is-culture-change

Rabig, J., Thomas, W., Kane, R. A., Cutler, L. J., & McAlilly, S. (2006). Radical redesign of nursing homes: Applying the Green House concept in Tupelo, Mississippi. *The Gerontologist, 46*(4), 533–539. https://doi
.org/10.1093/geront/46.4.533

Robert Wood Johnson Foundation. (2007). *"Green Houses" provide a small group setting alternative to nursing homes and a positive effect on residents' quality of life.*

Romaszewski, J. K. (2017). The journey to improving access to dental services for individuals in assisted living facilities across North Carolina. *North Carolina Medical Journal, 78*(6), 398–401. https://doi
.org/10.18043/ncm.78.6.398

Scope and Standards of Assisted Living Nursing Practice for Registered Nurses. (2006). www.alnursing.org

Shih, R. A., Acosta, J. D., Chen, E. K., Carbone, E. G., Xenakis, L., Adamson, D. M., & Chandra, A. (2018). Improving disaster resilience among older adults: Insights from public health departments and aging-in
-place efforts. *Rand Health Quarterly, 8*(1), 3. http://www.ncbi.nlm.nih.gov/pmc/articles/PMC6075802

Standards of Practice for Professional Chaplains in Long-term Care. (2012). https://professionalchaplains
.org/file/professional_standards_of_practice/sop_longtermcare.pdf

Stolee, P., Esbaugh, J., Aylward, S., Cathers, T., Harvey, D., Hillier, L., Keat, N., & Feightner, J. (2005). Factors associated with the effectiveness of continuing education in long-term care. *Gerontologist, 45*, 399–405.
https://doi.org/10.1093/geront/45.3.399

Stone, R. I., & Dawson, S. L. (2008). The origins of better jobs better care. *The Gerontologist, 48*, 5–13. https://
doi.org/10.1093/geront/48.Supplement_1.5

Stop. Think. Connect (2018a). *Department of Homeland Security*. Retrieved from https://stopthinkconnect
.org/resources/preview/tip-sheet-basic-tips-and-advice

Stop. Think. Connect (2018b). *Department of Homeland Security*. Retrieved from https://www.dhs.gov/sites/
default/files/publications/Cybersecurity%20for%20Older%20Americans_0.pdf

Tabloski, P. A. (2006). *Gerontological nursing*. Pearson Education.

Taylor, F. (1911). *The principles of scientific management.* http://strategy.sjsu.edu/www.stable/pdf/Taylor,%20 F.%20W.%20(1911).%20New%20York,%20Harper%20&%20Brothers.pdf

The Joint Commission. (2014). Joint Commission Perspectives, 34(1), 8–13.

Thomason, S., & Bernhardt, A. (2017). *California's homecare crisis: Raising wages is key to the solution.* UC Berkeley Center for Labor Research and Education. http://laborcenter.berkeley.edu/californias-homecare-crisis

Touhy, T. A., & Jett, K. (2018). *Ebersole & Hess' gerontological nursing and healthy aging* (5th ed). Elsevier.

U.S. Department of Health and Human Services and U.S. Department of Labor. (2003). *The future supply of long-term care workers in relation to the aging baby boom generation: Report to Congress.* Office of the Assistant Secretary for Planning and Evaluation. https://aspe.hhs.gov/basic-report/future-supply-long-term-care-workers-relation-aging-baby-boom-generation

U.S. Department of Labor. (n.d.). *Preparing the workplace for everyone: Implementation, communicating about and distributing the plan.* https://www.dol.gov/agencies/odep/publications/reports/preparing-the-workplace-for-everyone

U.S. General Accounting Office. (1999). *Assisted living: Quality of care and consumer protection issues* (GAO/T-HEHS-99-111).

Vega, C. P., & Bernarnd, A. (2016). *Interprofessional collaboration to improve health care: An introduction.* Medscape. www.medscape.com

Vespa, J. (2018). *The U.S joins other countries with large aging populations.* https://www.census.gov/library/stories/ 2018/03/graying-america.html

von Bertalanfy, L. (1968). *General system theory: Foundations, development, applications* (Rev. ed.). George Brazllier.

Wallace, S. P., Cochran, S. D., Durazo, E. M., & Ford, C. L. (2011). *The health of aging lesbian, gay and bisexual adults in California.* UCLA Center for Health Policy Research.

Walters, K. L., Evans-Canpbell, T., Simoni, J., Ronquillo, T., & Bhuyan, R. (2006). My spirit in my heart. Identity experiences and challenges among American Indian tow-spirit women. *Journal of Lesbian Studies, 10*(1/2) 125–149. https://doi.org/10.1300/J155v10n01_07

Weber, M. (1947). *The theory of social and economic organizations.* Oxford University Press.

Wilson, K. (2007). Historical evolution of assisted living in the United States: 1979 to the present. *The Gerontologist, 47,* 8–22. https://doi.org/10.1093/geront/47.supplement_1.8

Wolf, A. (2002). NFPA standards guide life safety for many assisted living facilities. *NFPA Journal,* 39–42. https://www.nfpa.org/News-andresearch/Publications

Wolfe, K. (2018). *Kaiser Permanente South San Francisco's groundbreaking home palliative care program receives prestigious honor.* https://everythingsouthcity.com/2018/04/kaiser-permanente-south-san-franciscos-groundbreaking-home-palliative-care-program-receives-prestigious-honor

Wunderlich, G., & Kohler, P. (Eds.). (2001). *Improving the quality of long-term care.* 27. National Academies Press. https://www.nia.nih.gov/health/what-long-term-care

Zimmerman, S., & Sloane, P. (2007). Definitions and classification of assisted living. *The Gerontologist, 47,* 33–39. https://doi.org/10.1093/geront/47.supplement_1.33Luptatur as accum quidita temque porestium

INDEX

Printed in the United States
by Baker & Taylor Publisher Services